MW01006162

Sex 101

*Getting Your Sex Life
Off to a Great Start*

CLIFFORD & JOYCE PENNER

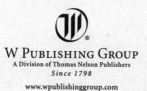

W PUBLISHING GROUP
A Division of Thomas Nelson Publishers
Since 1798

www.wpublishinggroup.com

Published by W Publishing Group, a division of Thomas Nelson, Inc., P.O. Box 141000, Nashville, Tennessee 37214.

Scripture references used in this book are from THE NEW KING JAMES VERSION. Copyright © 1979, 1980, 1982, Thomas Nelson, Inc., Publishers.

ISBN 0-8499-4510-0

Printed in the United States of America
04 05 06 07 08 QWM 5 4 3 2 1

CONTENTS

SO YOU'VE FOUND THE LOVE OF YOUR LIFE . . .

. . . and you're going to get married. Or perhaps you are newly-weds, and you're feeling all the newness and emotions created by joining your two families. For most of you these are very special days and months to remember. For all of you, they are exciting and life changing.

The two of you have made one of the most important decisions of your lives. This book is *not* about making that decision. It *is* about preparing for a great sex life in marriage once you have chosen each other as lifetime partners.

Perhaps you don't think you need any help in preparing for your sexual relationship as husband and wife. Some of you may be right. Not everyone needs to prepare in order to have a happy sex life in marriage. Some couples really can "do what comes naturally" and have a delightful, fulfilling experience. But for the majority, lack of preparation leads to sharp disappointment, even despair.

We've written this book to help you prepare, not just for your wedding night, but for a lifetime of exhilarating, satisfying, and nurturing sexual experiences.

To prepare when you don't need to is a happier mistake than not to prepare and find out you should have. Intelligent, deliberate preparation for sharing your lives together intimately will be a worthy investment you won't regret.

We were fortunate that our sex life in marriage got off to a great start and is a fulfilling, delightful part of our lives today. We are convinced that our successful beginning can be attributed to the knowledge and encouraging attitudes about sex in marriage that Joyce received during a Preparation for Marriage class she took right before we were married. Her eagerness to share that information with Cliff opened our communication about this vital dimension of our relationship. From our own positive experience and the changes we have observed in hundreds of couples' lives, we share the information in this book with an overwhelming conviction that accurate knowledge, healthy attitudes and expectations, and the ability for the two of you to talk openly about sex will significantly enhance your relationship. We have included discussion questions to help you and your partner share desires and expectations for your relationship. And we have also included, at the end of Chapters 2 through 7, common questions we have received in helping numerous couples prepare for marriage. We hope *Sex 101* will equip you with the tools to get your sex life off to a great start!

1 MAKE SEX SIZZLE

Sizzle pictures the intensity of a relationship. We might think of sizzle as the passion or excitement of sex. Passion can express itself in intense sexual feelings as well as anger or other emotions. Relationships with high passion are often both intensely sexual and emotionally volatile. Yet, most couples enjoy some level of sizzle, at least when they start out.

Passion is the flame of your sexual relationship. For some couples, passion ignited slowly while others experienced almost instant intensity. You may still be driven by that fervent excitement so common to a new relationship or you may have already made the transition from the intensity of a new attraction to a warm glow that can be sparked into a sizzle. We might make the comparison to lighting a fire. Depending on the type of firewood, some fires ignite almost instantly. Others are slow to get started. All fires eventually die down but can be kept alive if they are stoked and firewood is added before the last spark is out.

To encourage the spark in your sex life, be sure you give it the tending you would a fire that you want to keep burning. Encourage the excitement about being together. Avoid sameness, predictability, and boredom. Expand your ability to be vulnerable with each other—to let go and be out of control. Stretch yourselves to live life to the fullest. Inhibitions stifle passion. Insecurities, anxieties, distrust, guilt, hurt, and disappointments will dampen sizzle. Elements of suspense, intrigue, and newness accompanied with respect, honor, and care will nurture the spark of your sex life.

Whether you begin your married sex life as virgins or one or both of you have been sexually active prior to your marriage, the transition from premarital passion to a married sexual relationship is a critical one. It can contribute to—or hinder—the positive adjustment that brings the highest peaks of happiness that married life offers.

BE INTENTIONAL

Intentionality in your sex life will not only increase the quality of your times together, but also the quantity or frequency with which you enjoy each other. Sex is not something that happens to us and great sex will not just happen for you, but you can make your sex life great by being intentional about it. Be sure you save time and energy for each other. Take fifteen minutes a day to connect emotionally and spiritually. End those times with at least thirty seconds of passionate kissing. Plan for a weekly date night and/or a couple of hours to enjoy each other's bodies. Once a month, allow a day for just the two of you, and once a quarter, spend a weekend together undistracted.

COUNTER FALSE EXPECTATIONS

False expectations cause havoc and zap the spark. When he pictures it one way and she another, those differences must be clarified and negotiated. You will be talking about and clarifying your expectations as you read through the next chapter. Even that process can add fun and sizzle.

ELIMINATE DEMANDS

Sex by demand leads to sex without spark or to no sex at all. Freely give yourselves to each other. Never pressure each other. If either of you feels pressure, talk about it right away. The other one may not be aware of communicating pressure or triggering that in you.

HEAL FROM PAST HURTS

If either of you were raised in an alcoholic or emotionally out-of-control home, suffered sexual abuse or trauma, or were in a past destructive relationship, you will need to pursue help to undo those hurts. Often the impact of past hurts doesn't show up in a dating relationship, but surfaces quickly as marriage approaches or early in marriage. Free yourselves and your marriage bed from that baggage. If addictions control one of you, those will definitely need to be faced and managed in order for intimacy and passion to grow between the two of you.

HAVE FUN AND PLAY TOGETHER

Playfulness makes sex fun and rewarding for both spouses. Cuddling, holding, and caressing will set the stage for playfulness. Freedom and creativity are essential ingredients. If one of you is more likely to add the fun part, talk about which of you that would be and how to encourage that spouse to feel the freedom to lead.

PURSUE NEWNESS

A good place to begin is to vary the location and the setting or atmosphere of your sexual encounters. You can vary the room or the area of a room where you get together sexually. You can also experiment with lighting, the position in your bed, putting a comforter on the floor or by the fireplace. It will add spark if you take turns choosing the place and creating the setting.

KEEP THE PILOT LIGHT ON

Encourage sexual thoughts and feelings throughout the day and always turn those toward your spouse. Prepare yourself mentally for your sexual times. If your times are intentional and planned you can anticipate and prepare for each other. It is important for each of you to take responsibility to create the best conditions for sex. In other words, if you are more likely to feel passion when you are rested, don't leave sex for the last event of the night. If you are most sparked by privacy, be sure to have window coverings, door locks, and sound barriers. If you need talk time before you can allow intensity, plan that into your time together. Whatever you need, you are the one to make that happen. You are more likely to keep the pilot light on if you go to bed together and if you kiss passionately every day. So stay connected and keep kissing—your sex will have sizzle.

2 CLARIFY EXPECTATIONS

A fulfilling married sexual life is in part dependent on its start. Many couples have difficulty transferring their premarital passion into their marriages because they have false expectations about married sex, they lack accurate information, and they are unable to communicate openly about themselves and what each envisions as a healthy, fulfilling married sex life. Many of the couples who come to us for sexual therapy say their sexual problem started on their honeymoon or shortly thereafter. *Often the pain and disappointment could have been avoided if someone had talked with them openly about sex and taken the time to guide them through a process of discussing and negotiating their expectations for their sexual relationship in marriage.* That is what we hope to do for you in this chapter. Have fun as you read and talk through your expectations.

WHAT TURNS YOU ON?

A colleague of ours once said, "If you want to turn on a woman, talk to her. If you want to turn on a man, stroke him." Even though that is a big generalization, there is some truth in our friend's observation of the difference between men and women sexually. What is true for you?

Take turns finishing each of the following statements.

YOU AND ME

My first impression of you was _____.

What I like about you is _____.

My general image of you is _____.

What puzzles me about you is _____.

My most frequent daydreams about you are _____.

I love it when you _____.

I feel uncomfortable with you when _____.

When I am upset with you, I _____.

When you are upset with me, I _____.

I worry about you most when _____.

Our physical involvement makes me feel _____.

The best feeling in any physical, sexual contact is _____.

I feel sexual sensations when _____.

When I fantasize about sex, I picture _____.

What turns me on is _____.

The surest turnoff for me is _____.

What I think you need to know about me is _____.

When I imagine having sex with you, I feel _____.

When I think of our future, I _____.

What works for you sexually will continue to change, grow, and develop throughout your marriage. Continue talking about your sexual feelings, needs, and desires. Plan into your marriage a yearly review of this "What Turns You On?" section.

YOUR SEXUAL PATTERNS

To whatever degree you are physical with each other, you will have established certain patterns. Talk about those patterns with one another.

Sexual Desire

Becoming one sexually begins with sexual desire. All of us are created with that urge.

- How often do you feel the urge to be touched and to be close or for sexual arousal and release?
- What stimulates those urges in you?
- How do you handle those urges?
- What changes have you noticed in your sexual desire since you started dating?

Initiation

Initiation is acting upon your desire.

- How do you handle your desire (e.g., ignore it, substitute physical exercise, call a friend, pray, masturbate, or express it with each other)?

- If you act on the desire with each other, who initiates that action?
- How do you express that desire to each other?
- Are you happy with how that happens?
- Is it mutual?
- What about your response to your sexual desire would you like to change?
- What about your partner's response to his/her sexual desire would you like to change?

Pleasure

Pleasure is the process of enjoying one another. To what degree have the two of you been or are you currently physically involved with each other? Circle any behaviors on the list below.

Hand-holding
Hugging
Polite kissing
Total-mouth kissing
Intense, passionate kissing
Full-body rubbing with clothes on
Breast stimulation over clothes
Genital stimulation over clothes
Breast stimulation under clothes
Genital stimulation under clothes
Full-body pleasuring, no clothes
Oral-genital stimulation

Total sexual experience, except entry

Total sexual experience, including entry but without orgasm while inside

Total sexual experience, including entry and thrusting to ejaculation

- Does your involvement agree or disagree with your beliefs?
- If it agrees, is that mutual?
- If it disagrees or is not mutual, how might you change or get control of your sexual activity without shutting down your desires for one another? List behavioral changes that you could make. (For example, plan your times alone so that you could be interrupted and set clearly agreed-upon boundaries.)
- Do you experience discomfort, guilt, or inhibitions when you are engaged in physical touching with each other?
- If so, discuss how you might manage your times together to reduce or eliminate any negatives connected with your physical interaction.
- What kind of touching is most pleasurable to you?
- Are you aware of experiencing any arousal?
- Are you aware of any restrictions you have on allowing yourself sexual pleasure other than the decisions you have made to limit your sexual involvement before marriage?
- What events, feelings, or actions have contributed to your times of greatest pleasure without violation of your boundaries?

Letting Go

Letting go is the releasing of sexual intensity.

- Are you a person who needs control in your life, or are you able to let go and take risks?
- Have you ever experienced sexual release?
- If so, through what forms of stimulation?
- If not, has that been by decision or because of inhibition?
- What expectations do you have for sexual release and satisfaction in marriage?

Affirmation

- What do you feel after a time of being close physically?
- What do you need from your partner at that time?
- How might you express your affirmation of your partner?
- What affirmation would you expect as part of a total sexual experience once you are married?

YOUR BODIES

A woman who attended one of our premarital classes said, "I've never really liked my body. How do I bring this up to my fiancé before the honeymoon? I'd like to talk about it, but I don't know how."

How you feel about your body will affect how openly you will be able to share yourself, how freely you will be able to soak in the pleasure of your spouse's touch, and how enthusiastically you will go after sexual pleasure for yourself. If you do not feel good about yourself, you will have a hard time giving to or caring for someone else.

Your body image is your attitude about your body, especially your bodily appearance. Everyone would like to have that "perfect" figure or physique. Women are often concerned that their breasts are too big, too small, too flabby, too far apart, or too whatever. Men are concerned with the size of their penises, worrying that a smaller penis means they are less of a man and thus less likely to be able to satisfy a woman. The truth is that, despite all the Internet ads, the size of breasts or penises is unrelated to sexual pleasure or satisfaction.

Some people are generally dissatisfied with their appearance; others are unhappy with their weight. Still others struggle with how they are proportioned.

If you are fairly accepting of your body and if your view of your body matches your ideal, you have a good body image. Body-image problems occur when there is a large gap between how you view your body and what you see as ideal. If the way you would like to look is different from the way you think you do look, you will have difficulty accepting yourself and will probably have difficulty being free with your body sexually. If that is the case, what can you do to bridge the gap? How can you bring your view of yourself closer to your ideal?

The first step toward body-image enhancement is to examine your view of yourself. Is how you see yourself consistent with how others see you? When you talked about your body with your partner, did his or her feedback affirm your view of yourself? If not, what has contributed to your inability to accept and appreciate your body the way it is? Past sexual abuse, childhood physical abuse, a painful illness, and lack of warm touch and holding during infancy all contribute to a poor body image. Negative verbal messages about your body from peers, parents, or other respected adults may have contributed to a poor body image. You may need your spouse's ongoing affirmation, both verbally and through touching, to mend those past hurts. You might spend some time in front of a mirror each day, thanking God for having designed you the way He did.

The second step in bringing your own body view closer to that of your ideal is to determine ways you can change your body. There are many different ways this can be done. Losing or gaining weight and exercising are the most commonly pursued options. Women may also use makeup and different hairstyles; men may choose to shave or not shave and vary their haircut. Both partners can vary their choice of clothing, straighten or correct faulty teeth, or improve their posture; ultimately even plastic surgery is an option.

The third and final suggestion for bringing your ideal closer to your real view of yourself is to reevaluate your ideal. What are you measuring yourself against? Who are your models? Are you looking at the extremes held up by the media? How do these "ideal" images compare with the significant and valued people in your life? If your expectations are so far out of reach that you will always feel dissatisfied, we recommend the following process: Commit yourself to one other person who will hold you accountable to get rid of the current ideals and start selecting more realistic body models. If your new models are people with whom you can talk freely, ask them how they achieved their physical condition.

The struggle to feel good about your body is a process of becoming open with yourself and your partner. This includes honesty concerning your feelings about yourself, feeling comfortable being in the nude, caring for your body, and allowing yourself to receive validation through touch and verbal feedback from others in your world. A sense of comfort with and acceptance of your body will contribute to freedom and pleasure in your sexual experiences. Compare your views of yourselves with each other.

YOUR EXPECTATIONS

Take time to fantasize together about your ideal sexual experience in marriage. Even though you may not have thought about it, you probably have a picture of your ideal sexual experience.

What do you envision happening between the two of you and inside each of you during deeply satisfying lovemaking? When do you expect to have your first sexual time together on your honeymoon? When and where will it happen? Who will initiate? Do you imagine that experience will lead to intercourse? How often do you expect to have sexual times on your honeymoon? What about after the honeymoon? What percentage of those sexual times together will lead to intercourse? What parts of your current physical involvement would you like to continue after marriage? Which ones would you hope to change?

What expectations do you have of each other, generally and sexually? Take time to list ten expectations you have for your spouse. Then, across from each expectation, identify how you would be affected if your spouse did not fulfill these expectations.

Share these with each other and talk about creative ways to meet your expectations without putting negative demands or pressure on either of you. *Demands stifle; giving softens.* Practice giving to each other without demand.

YOUR SEXUAL PAST

The two of you bring to your sexual relationship unique past experiences. Your families will have modeled and communicated different views of sexuality. Understanding those differences and your uniqueness will be essential to knowing each other sexually. You may have sexual secrets that seem very risky to share. You may still suffer the consequences of past hurts. It is completely understandable that you might feel hesitant to talk about your sexual past. You may worry about the effect your revelations will have on your partner. That is a realistic concern. In fact, you may want to discuss your decision with a counselor before you take that step.

YOUR DIFFERENCES

Although the wife wants to be sexually satisfied by her husband, this desire is awakened in her long after she has discovered that she loves him enough to die for him, while a man on the other hand desires to possess a woman physically long before he cares sufficiently to raise his little finger for her. That the love of a woman normally comes from the soul to the senses . . . forms one of the chief differences between the two, and often leads to the greatest misunderstanding.[1]

In our culture, emotional intimacy seems to be something women need much more than men. Women tend to feel the desire for sex when they feel connected with their husbands, while men tend to feel connected as the result of a positive sexual experience. The most common stereotypes in our culture are that men "play" at love to get sex and women "play" at sex to get love. "Briefly stated, love is linked to self-esteem in women. For a man, romantic experiences with his wife are warm and enjoyable and memorable—but not necessary. For a woman, they are her lifeblood. Her confidence, her sexual response, and her zest for living are often directly related to those tender moments when she feels deeply loved and appreciated by her man."[2]

You may or may not relate to these findings that describe men and women. What is important is that the two of you plan for *your* differences and understand some common issues that are gender unique. Some differences between men and women that affect sexual relationships are reported to us regularly. Which of the differences on the following list are true for you? You may have additional differences to add to the list.

Male/Female Differences

He likes the room cold.	She likes the room hot.
He is result oriented.	She is process oriented.
He wants to solve her problem.	She wants him to listen to her problem.

He wants sex.	She wants romance.
He wants to engage in activities.	She wants to talk.
He likes intense kissing.	She likes pliable kisses.
Sexually, he goes for more.	Sexually, less makes her hungry for more.

A great resource for dealing with male/female differences is John Gray's book *Men Are from Mars, Women Are from Venus.*[3]

Knowing what is a turn-on for you and your partner, being clear about each of your visions of a positive sexual encounter, and understanding, accepting, and adapting to your male/female differences are positive ways you can validate each other's expectations for your married sex life. The intimacy that will develop between the two of you as you pursue this process of determining and maintaining clear expectations will be a key to a great sex life.

■ ■ ■

Why should I have to learn about sex? Can't I just do what comes naturally?

If we lived in a primitive society and started experimenting sexually from the time we felt any sexual awareness, we might know what to do naturally. In primitive societies we might also be "initiated" by an older person of the opposite sex. Because of our Christian and moral values, however, it is inappropriate that we practice such experimenting and initiation rituals. Nor do we watch others have intercourse unless we watch distorted sexual encounters on television and in movies.

Thus, the only way you can learn how to enjoy a satisfying sexual relationship in marriage is to educate yourselves, teach each other, and learn with each other. Whether or not your childhood or dating experiences have prepared you to easily find sexual pleasure and satisfaction, you can *learn* to be a good lover!

I've never had sex before, and I'm afraid my wife is going to be disappointed with my lack of knowledge.

Talk about your concern and learn together. Just as you don't get a quality education by reading the first page of several different books, you do not become a competent lover by repeating the same inadequate experiences over and over. You become a competent lover by listening to each other's guidance and learning through years of intimate sharing with the same person. The greatest sexual fulfillment comes for those who learn and grow throughout a lifetime commitment to each other.

In movies and TV men are portrayed as ready, willing, and assertive, and women are passive and available. Is there any truth to this?

This myth produces incredible demand! It demands that the husband behave as though he is interested even when he is not. It demands that the wife be responsive to her husband's arousal even when she is not interested. Even though both can decide to participate in a sexual time together when one is feeling the desire and the other is not, it should not be by demand. Sex should always be a choice. Demand is a killer to a healthy, long-term sexual relationship.

While there are typical gender differences between men and women, women can learn to be assertive and men can learn to be sensitive. Men do tend to be more competitive, assertive, and rational, and are often not as aware of their feelings as women are. Women tend to be more gentle, nurturing, intuitive, emotionally responsive, and relationally oriented. All men and all women exhibit some portion of all of these qualities. Breaking away from these traditional role expectations is often beneficial to a couple's relationship.

If you develop your potential in the areas of expression that are not as natural for you, your sexual life will be enhanced. As men learn to know, share, and be sensitive to feelings, and as women become more assertive in expressing their sexual desires, needs, and wishes, their capacity for ecstasy is heightened.

Real men truly become "real men" as they discover and develop their romantic and intimacy capabilities. Sensitivity is a positive male attribute!

3 KNOW YOUR BODY

Your sexual organs and their functioning during the sexual experience comprise an awesome and beautiful system. The intricate details of this sexual response have been measured by Masters and Johnson and categorized into four phases: excitement, plateau, orgasmic, and resolution.

These responses may occur due to sexual intercourse; to manual, oral, or self-stimulation of the genitals; intense hugging; deep kissing; petting; fantasy; visual input; or any love play. Sexual intercourse is not necessary for full sexual release, nor does sexual intercourse guarantee full sexual release. This is vital information, especially for understanding the difference between sexual feelings and behavior as it relates to your sexual decisions and responsibility.

As you read the following discussion of what happens in your bodies during each of the four phases of the sexual response pattern, note any of the responses you are aware of or assume have happened to you. Also note any of the responses that you believe are difficult for you or have not happened. Share your thoughts with each other.

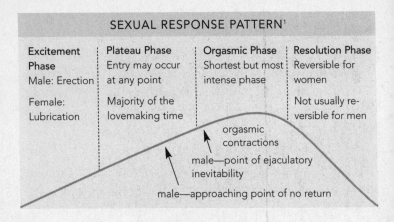

SEXUAL RESPONSE PATTERN[1]

Excitement Phase	Plateau Phase	Orgasmic Phase	Resolution Phase
Male: Erection	Entry may occur at any point	Shortest but most intense phase	Reversible for women
Female: Lubrication	Majority of the lovemaking time		Not usually reversible for men

orgasmic contractions

male—point of ejaculatory inevitability

male—approaching point of no return

THE EXCITEMENT PHASE—AROUSAL

The excitement phase, the first stage of the sexual response pattern, occurs involuntarily without any stimulation when you are relaxed or asleep. The excitement phase may precede sexual desire—the urge to be close physically or to be stimulated sexually—but is more likely to result from stimulation. For both the man and the woman, the changes of the excitement phase are due to vasocongestion (blood and fluid rushing into the sexual organs).

Female Excitement

The clitoris is most important for the woman during the excitement phase. It becomes engorged with blood the same way the penis does. It doubles or triples in size as blood and fluid rush into its venous spaces.

The clitoris, the only organ in the human anatomy designed

solely for receiving and transmitting sexual stimuli, confirms that God designed women to be intensely sexual beings, not just "vaginas" that are recipients of the man's sexual aggression. Physiologically, pleasure is the clitoris's only function. The woman, not the man, was created with the clitoris. Consider this fact very seriously as you begin your sexual life together. It should affect how you make love, how the woman feels about herself as a sexual being, and how the man relates to her sexually. Couples who are aware of the unique importance of the clitoris rarely fall into the "passive woman versus aggressive man" mentality that leaves the woman unfulfilled in the sexual act and the man unhappy with the woman's lack of involvement.

Intense pleasure and pain are closely related in our bodies. Those areas, such as the clitoris, that are loaded with nerve endings are most receptive to pleasure and, for the same reason, most receptive to pain. As the woman's arousal moves to intense pleasure, the clitoris becomes so sensitive she can readily experience clitoral pain, especially if the stimulation is directly on the head of the clitoris, too intense, or continues too long. That is why it is vital to understand that most women prefer stimulation *around* the clitoris rather than directly on the head. Most women also prefer the stimulation to vary in intensity, and they respond better if their arousal is allowed to build in waves with intermittent, rather than continuous, stimulation of the clitoris. A lighter, teasing touch satisfies most. Ultimately what works best is if the woman is the authority on her own body and guides her husband in clitoral touch. There is no way he can automatically know what is going to be most pleasurable.

During the excitement phase, other changes happen in the woman's body. The labia minora (inner lips) become engorged and extend outward while the labia majora (outer lips) spread flat as if the genital area is opening up to receive the penis. As the arousal builds, the woman's genitals take on a slight funnel shape in preparation for penile entry.

Internally, the uterus begins to pull up and away from the vagina; this pulls the cervix out of the way so the penis will not strike against it during thrusting. However, this preparation does not occur when the woman has a tipped uterus; the cervix does not get out of the way of the penis. That is why it can be struck, causing a sharp, stabbing pain during deep thrusting.

The vagina lubricates within twenty seconds of any form of sexual stimulation. The lubrication is secreted like beads of per-spiration along the wall of the vagina to make the entry of the penis into the vagina a smooth and comfortable activity. Even though lubrication is the sign of *physical* readiness, only the woman can determine when she is *emotionally* ready for entry. The involuntary response of lubrication cannot be triggered by will or determination. Anxiety or pressure to perform is likely to hinder lubrication, so during your sexual encounters we recom-mend using a lubricant. Many different lubricants are available. K-Y Jelly is water-based, so it dries easily but is latex compatible. Albolene (a facial cleanser) is very good but not recommended for use with a diaphragm or condom. Natural oils are also popu-lar. Products designed especially for sexual intercourse that will not interfere with the effectiveness of condoms and diaphragms include Probe, Liquid Silk, Astroglide, and many others.

The breasts also change during the initial excitement phase; nipple erection is the most obvious response, and general engorgement causes a slight increase in breast size. The areola, the area around the nipple, usually darkens and becomes slightly engorged, especially as the woman's excitement intensifies. We have received letters from engaged women who were concerned about this change in their nipples as they became aroused or felt chilled. They wondered if this change in their nipples would be negative for their husbands. On the contrary, men are usually excited by the woman's nipple erection.

Male Excitement

The penis is the primary receiver and transmitter of sexual sensations in the man. The penile response of erection is parallel to clitoral engorgement and vaginal lubrication in the woman. It is that involuntary response that occurs throughout the day and night and can be brought about by sexual thoughts or by direct or indirect stimulation of the penis itself. Erection is necessary for intercourse, so men who have had difficulty with arousal or loss of erection worry about their ability to respond.

Erections can easily be interrupted by negative or nonsexual stimulation such as the telephone ringing, a loud noise, a negative thought, a special concern, a harsh word, or a critical comment. Erections can be lost and regained when relaxation and freedom allow that response. This is likely to happen during extended love play, yet erections can also be maintained for extended periods of time without ejaculation. The latter is most likely to occur when the stimulation is varied and the intensity of the experience flows in waves.

In addition to the penis becoming erect as blood and fluid rush into it, the scrotum thickens and elevates slightly. The man, as well as the woman, may experience a sexual flush in the upper third of the body. Nipple erection occurs in about 60 percent of men.

THE PLATEAU PHASE

The plateau phase is the phase that varies most in length; it can last a few minutes or continue for hours. It all depends on how quickly each individual responds and what the couple desires. The plateau phase includes all the bodily changes that happen from the time of arousal until orgasm.

The changes that occur during the plateau phase are due to the buildup of tension and increased congestion in the genitals. When a long, extended period of love play occurs, this buildup of intensity will usually result in repeated waves of heightened arousal and then relaxation. They may continue as long as the partners give each other and themselves the freedom to ride these waves; then the intensity with one of the waves will build to the point of automatically triggering an orgasm.

Male Plateau

Externally, the penis becomes slightly more engorged and deeper in color during the plateau phase while the glans, or head, of the penis increases in diameter. The scrotum also thickens and elevates more. Fluid containing sperm may seep from the penis during the plateau phase before the point of ejaculation; that is why withdrawal of the penis from the vagina before ejaculation is not a reliable method of birth control.

Internally during this phase the testes enlarge 50 to 100 percent. The right testicle rises and rotates a quarter turn. Near the end of the plateau phase as the man nears the point of orgasm, three changes warn him that he is about to ejaculate. The left testicle rises and rotates a quarter turn, the prostate gland contracts, and the sphincter from the bladder shuts off so no seminal fluid will be forced into the bladder and no urine will be expelled during ejaculation. No man can identify these specific changes, thinking, for example, *There goes the left one,* but he *can* sense that he is about to ejaculate. The seminal fluid is traveling to the base of the penis.

Once these changes have occurred, the process is in motion. The man is approaching ejaculatory inevitability, the point of no return (see graph, p. 20). He *will* ejaculate! If a man wishes to learn to delay his ejaculation, he must gain control *prior* to these physical changes.

Female Plateau

As the sexual experience progresses, more and more is happening internally for the woman, and less is occurring externally. This fact symbolizes women's more internal experience, in contrast to men's more external, obvious response.

The slight external changes include the increase in size and brightening in color of the labia minora a minute or two before orgasm. The Bartholin's gland just inside the labia secretes one to three drops of a substance designed to enhance impregnation by changing the pH balance of the vagina. At the same time, the clitoral glans retracts under the clitoral hood, allowing more direct stimulation.

Internally, many significant changes must occur for the woman before her intensity will be strong enough to trigger an orgasm. The uterus, which began to elevate during the excitement phase, now elevates even more. The nonerotic upper two-thirds of the vagina expands or balloons to hold the seminal fluid for impregnation; this area is known as the *seminal pool*. The outer third of the vagina becomes intensely engorged to form the orgasmic platform. Some women are aware of the pleasurable vaginal grasping response as arousal during the plateau phase intensifies. These bodily changes verify that the woman's sexual response was designed for both reproduction and pleasure.

Male and Female Transition from Plateau to Orgasm

The specific changes that happen for both men and women during the transition from plateau to orgasm usually go relatively unnoticed. There is the involuntary extension of the foot called the *carpopedal spasm*. Both the heart rate and the blood pressure increase. Involuntary pelvic thrusting occurs as arousal approaches orgasm, and general muscular tension builds with spasticlike contractions.

More obvious changes also occur. The skin flushes in the chest, neck, and face—almost a blushing effect due to the widespread vasocongestion. Facial grimaces are common because of the involuntary contracting of the facial muscles. Gasping or moaning responses are due in part to hyperventilation (heavy breathing), which is virtually inevitable and necessary for both men and women in order to be able to orgasm. Women who have difficulty with orgasm usually stop these intense gasping, grimacing, and breathing responses because they feel self-conscious. Yet these changes are necessary for both men and women to make the transition from the plateau phase to the orgasmic response, and men enjoy these responses in their wives.

THE ORGASMIC PHASE

The orgasmic phase is the shortest and most intense of the four phases. It is a reflex response that lasts only a few seconds. You cannot choose to respond with an orgasm as you can choose to bend your elbow, but you can control or inhibit the response by stopping the natural, involuntary responses in your body. Or you can enhance the possibility of an orgasmic response by becoming active and pursuing genital stimulation—penile thrusting for the man and clitoral and/or vaginal stimulation for the woman.

As the intensity builds, the tension increases to the point at which the orgasmic reflex is set off. The autonomic, or involuntary, nervous system has switched control from the relaxed branch (the parasympathetic) to the active, fight-or-flight branch (the sympathetic). Thus, the more active you are, the more your body is encouraged to respond orgasmically (which is usually what the woman needs); and the quieter and more passive you are, the more your response is slowed down (which is usually what the man needs). Since orgasm is a reflex, a person who actively receives enough stimulation will eventually be orgasmic.

Female Orgasm

All the significant orgasmic changes in the woman take place internally. Because those responses are not obvious, there has been much confusion about women's orgasmic response.

Internally, the woman has two centers of orgasmic response, the uterus and the vagina. The uterus contracts similarly to the way it contracts during the early stages of labor. (This is why doctors rule out orgasm when a woman is threatening to miscarry or go into early labor.) Sometimes women resist these contractions because they are experienced as slightly painful, but as women learn to focus on the intense pleasure of the contractions, they become highly enjoyable. Intense pleasure and pain are so close that the switch from one to the other is very possible. The second internal response center is the outer third of the vagina—the orgasmic platform. The contractions of the PC (pubococcygeus) muscle that surrounds both the vagina and the rectal sphincter occur eight-tenths of a second apart, with three to five contractions in a mild orgasm and eight to twelve contractions in a more intense orgasm. These uterine and vaginal responses happen simultaneously.

Because the clitoris is retracted completely under the hood during orgasm, the woman may need very direct clitoral stimulation at that particular time. She can develop signals to communicate that need to her husband.

Male Orgasm

The man's orgasm is experienced in two stages. In the first stage, the internal genitalia respond a few seconds before ejaculation. The contractions of these internal structures—the seminal duct system, the prostate gland, the rectal sphincter, and the urinary bladder—occur at intervals of eight-tenths of a second just as they do in the woman. These contractions move the ejaculate to the base of the penis, preparing it for the ejaculation.

During stage two, the seminal fluid carrying the sperm is expelled. This is the ejaculation. Having reached this point of ejaculatory inevitability, nothing can stop this response; it is, indeed, inevitable. The contractions at the base of the penis that cause the expulsion of the seminal fluid also occur at intervals of eight-tenths of a second. For the average male, a standard ejaculation contains 3.5 to 5 cubic centimeters of ejaculate (about 1 teaspoon) and 175 to 500 million spermatozoa.

Orgasmic Differences Between Men and Women

Women's orgasmic responses seem to differ greatly from one experience to another and from one woman to another. Men seem to be more similar in their orgasmic responses. This may be due to the wide range of the contractions during orgasm for women (from three to twelve) and their capacity for having more than one orgasm.

Women have a physiologically unlimited potential for orgasms; they are limited only by their desire, their pursuit, and their stamina. In contrast, men, except for a very small percentage, need a refractory period of at least twenty minutes—and usually hours—before they can regain arousal, erection, and ejaculation.

As a man ages, the refractory period increases. It also seems that the more frequently a man ejaculates, the longer it takes until he is able to be restimulated.

Even though women have unlimited potential for orgasms, many women struggle to even experience one. And not all women desire more than one response. Some women have extended orgasms. These are orgasms that come one right after another with no refractory period. Other women have multiple or sequential orgasms. These women respond orgasmically, have a slight refractory period, then respond again with another orgasm.

The woman's orgasm can be interrupted at any point; the man's cannot. Once the man has reached the point of ejaculatory inevitability, nothing can be done to stop it; the reflex is in motion. Because of this irreversibility, women have often been taught they should not arouse a man because once a man is aroused he cannot control his behavior. This just is not true! Men are responsible for their own sexual behavior just as women are. Ejaculatory control—learning to gain control *before* the point of no return—is a separate issue that also *can* be learned.

The longer the time between sexual releases, the greater the difference between men and women's timing of sexual response. If the sexual experience is the first one in a long time, a woman will tend to be slower in her response and will experience less intensity in her release, while a man will tend to be quicker in his arousal and release and experience more buildup and intensity. We believe this tendency—to go in the opposite direction—is one more indication that couples were designed to be together and to experience sexual release on a regular basis.

While women experience difficulty with and pressure to be orgasmic (the active phase of the sexual response cycle), men's pressure is with getting or keeping erections (the passive phase of the sexual response cycle) or with ejaculating too quickly. This is likely because men tend to be active during sex and women tend to be passive. If you wish to prevent these difficulties, both of you would do well to learn to enjoy both passively receiving pleasure and actively pursuing pleasure.

THE RESOLUTION PHASE

During this final phase of the sexual response, the body returns to its unstimulated state. Both the man and the woman experience the sensation of tension loss due to the release of engorgement and the diminishing of vasocongestion.

Male Resolution

In the male, the most obvious sign of resolution is the lessening of his erection. For most men, the full, firm erection will diminish immediately, but it may take some time for the penis to return to its prestimulated, flaccid state. A question that was asked during a premarital class relates to this issue: "Is it possible to stay hard after ejaculation, continue making love, and ejaculate again?" A few men report the ability to do that, and sexual therapists Alan and Donna Brauer, in their book *ESO,* suggest possible ways to enhance that possibility.[2] We would discourage a focus on reaching this goal, especially early in your sexual life. Goals such as this usually take away from the pleasure and create demand.

During resolution, some men experience heightened sensitivity, even pain, on the glans of the penis. If you should find that to be true for you, rather than draw away from your wife and leave her feeling rejected, inform her of this sensitivity and your need not to have any penile touching after ejaculation. You can hold and affirm each other without penile contact.

Men often feel relaxed and fall asleep quickly after an orgasm. This can be frustrating to the woman who may come down off her orgasm more slowly and desire a time of intimacy through conversation and touch. On the other hand, if the woman has experienced an intense orgasm or enough orgasmic release she, too, may fall asleep quickly.

Female Resolution

If the woman has been aroused but has not experienced release, she may feel the continued tension or engorgement for some time after the sexual experience. This can be frustrating for the woman, sometimes causing involuntary crying.

From a physiological perspective, we understand this crying to be the body's way of releasing the tension that did not get released orgasmically. Crying triggers the parasympathetic-nervous-system dominance, which helps the woman relax. When the couple can hold each other and share this crying release, the woman will eventually become more comfortable letting go with her husband and be able to allow an orgasmic release.

After an orgasm, the woman's clitoris returns to its pre-stimulated size within five to ten minutes. It takes about the same time for the labia minora and labia majora to return to their unstimulated size, position, and color. The uterus drops back into its original position relatively quickly after orgasm. The vaginal wall collapses within five to eight minutes while the congestion in the outer third of the vagina disappears in seconds.

When the woman has not had an orgasm, it will take longer for all of these changes to occur because the engorgement is released gradually. There have been no contractions to trigger the release. The greater the number of contractions, the more quickly the woman's body returns to its prestimulated state. During the resolution phase, you have the opportunity to affirm your intimacy regardless of the physical fulfillment that has been experienced. Some couples like to fall asleep together, others like to talk and cuddle, and still others like to get up and do something active together. Discover together what you enjoy. If your desires for handling the resolution time are different, negotiate those differences: One time go his way, another time her way, and sometimes compromise on both ways.

■ ■ ■

Why do some couples have simultaneous orgasms and some don't? Isn't that the best kind of sex?

Simultaneous orgasms are far from necessary for a fully satisfying sexual relationship, and striving for that goal will cause more trouble than it is worth, creating one of those demands that destroy pleasure. A husband and wife may incidentally orgasm at the same time, particularly if the wife has more than one orgasm, but it often is more enjoyable to orgasm separately and enjoy the intensity of each other's experience.

How does a woman know if she has had an orgasm?

Usually you will know by how you feel afterward. When you have had release, you feel the relaxation after the buildup of the sexual tension in your body. If not, you will feel the frustration or alertness of not having had release. An orgasm is basically a pelvic sneeze. Consider how you feel when your nasal passages are congested and you need to sneeze but you can't. That is the same feeling that occurs in the pelvic area when you have gotten aroused but have not had an orgasm. Another analogy shared by a person in one of our classes is that an orgasm can feel like opening up a well-shaken can of soda. However, we might add that orgasms are not always that intense.

Can a man stimulate a woman in such a way that she will always have an orgasm?

No, it is not the man's responsibility to assure a woman of an orgasm. There are definitely techniques he can learn that will be more enjoyable for her than others. The woman has to learn about her body and teach her husband what she needs to become stimulated. She also has to learn to be active in going after the stimulation she desires. In turn, he has to learn to enjoy her body for his pleasure without focusing on whether he is producing a response. His focus on her response will produce demand, not an orgasm.

What if the woman cannot have an orgasm during intercourse?

Although any woman can learn to be orgasmic during intercourse, if that's what she desires, the majority of women do not have orgasms during intercourse. Most women respond orgasmically to manual and/or clitoral stimulation. There are other women who respond during intercourse and still others who respond either way. Orgasmic response during intercourse can be stimulated by touching the clitoris or by stimulating the G-spot, an area in the vagina just beyond the pubococcygeus (PC) muscle toward the front of the woman's body. All variations are delightful ways of receiving sexual pleasure and release and have nothing to do with rightness or sexual maturity. What is right is what works for you!

If you have never had an orgasm, how do you get one?

There are entire books written on this topic. The one we recommend is *Becoming Orgasmic* by Julia Heiman and Joseph LoPiccolo.[3] We also have outlined a whole process for that purpose in our book *Restoring the Pleasure*.[4] Basically, there are four simple steps: stop trying, focus on pleasure, reduce self-consciousness, and get active. The goal you can set for yourself is to enjoy longer times of arousal and higher peaks of arousal. Eventually the orgasmic reflex will be triggered.

What if the woman hasn't reached orgasm and the man gets to the point of no return?

The man can continue to stimulate the woman after he ejaculates. Or the two of you can prevent this from happening by enjoying a longer time of stimulating the woman both before and during intercourse and teaching the man to delay ejaculation. All of these are satisfactory options.

4 DESIGN A SUCCESSFUL HONEYMOON

The fond memories of our happy honeymoon have lingered with us now for forty years. As it was for us, your honeymoon will be a special time just for the two of you. After the hustle and bustle of all the planning, and after the delightful celebration of your wedding with friends and relatives, this will be your time to relish those fond memories, cherish each other, and anticipate your future together.

You are the two people who will create the atmosphere that will make your honeymoon a success. It might rain the entire week even though you choose the Kona Coast on the big island of Hawaii, where the rainfall is only six inches per year. One of you could be sick. Your luggage could get lost. One of you could forget your passports. You could discover you did not have a reservation at the motel you thought was confirmed for your first night. Most couples feel fatigued as their honeymoon begins; you may feel completely wiped out.

Disappointments need not interfere with this joyous time in your life. How you deal with the unexpected can add to, rather than distract from, your blissful getaway. We are convinced that *you* can make your honeymoon an experience that you remember fondly, even if there are disappointments and adjustments that must be made.

What makes a honeymoon successful? Your fantasy might be never leaving your room because you are so exhausted from the sexual activity you are both enjoying. You may dream of being together nonstop. But if that is not your spouse's expectation, you may be sorely disappointed. You may be a couple who enjoys traveling together to new and exciting places. On the contrary, you may both look forward to a time of peace and quiet after all the busyness of the wedding. Only *you* can design the honeymoon that is right for the two of you! So use the information in this chapter only as it contributes to what will bring the greatest joy, fulfillment, and contentment to the two of you.

HONEYMOON CHOICES

The honeymoon is a time of transition from singleness into marriage. It is a time to enjoy each other without outside demands. Usually this works best when you make choices that allow for privacy, unhurriedness, and freedom from scheduled expectations or interruptions.

The First Twenty-four Hours

Many couples err when they try to cram too much into their first twenty-four hours together. The reception may end later than they expected; then they may have a long distance to travel to their first-night hotel. They may have invested in an expensive honeymoon suite but get to it after midnight and have to rush out in the morning to catch a flight to their ultimate honeymoon destination. They may hardly remember that first night because they were exhausted when they arrived, their anticipatory anxiety was high, and they were pressured to pack up and leave in the morning. When this happens, the couple certainly does not get to enjoy what they paid for. Careful planning of your time from the end of the reception and on can make a major difference for your entire honeymoon. *Remember: the honeymoon starts when you drive away from the reception!*

Whether you spend your first night at a modest local motel or a three-room penthouse suite, you should anticipate your special needs and desired circumstances. This will often be more important for the woman since she will have borne the greater burden during the wedding planning and events. And women tend to be more affected than men by the circumstances of what is supposed to be a romantic time. Thus, the woman's needs should be given top priority. Nevertheless, both of you need to be aware of what will make the first night special for you.

There are several issues to consider in planning the first twenty-four hours of your honeymoon. The first is *transportation*. Do you want to drive yourselves or have someone else drive when you leave the reception? If someone else will drive, who do you want that to be? The second consideration is *food*. Often the bridal couple does very little eating at the reception. You might arrange with the person in charge of food for your reception to have a food basket packed for you to take along as you leave. It can be a fun connecting time to have a picnic in your room when you arrive.

The third consideration is *timing*. Allow more time than you think you need from the end of the reception until you leave for your honeymoon destination the next day.

The fourth is *clothing and personal items*. Consider what you want to wear when you leave the reception, what you will need to get ready for spending the night, and what you will need for the next morning. Have those items packed separately from the rest of your honeymoon luggage. That way you will not have to spend your time packing and repacking. If you don't want to take the first-night items with you on the rest of the honeymoon, arrange for a friend or family member to pick them up from the hotel desk after you leave.

Other plans might include any of your personal preferences. For example, if one of you dislikes certain color schemes, you might ask about the room decor at your honeymoon hotel. Others have fears of heights or feeling closed in. Temperature may need to be anticipated; you might arrange to have the heater or the air conditioner turned on in your room before you arrive. Be aware of who each of you are and what would add to the pleasantness of your first night together as a married couple.

Connecting Time

The purpose of the honeymoon is to provide connection between the two of you. The honeymoon conditions should help do that. In what situations have you felt most connected? What kind of setting has pulled you away from each other?

You may just love to spend time together. Outside activities may not be essential to your enjoyment. On the other hand, you may do better with a balance of together time, alone time, and activity time. Eating out or taking walks together may be good for you. Having a project may be a way the two of you can connect. You may want to take along your gift list and write thank-you notes together. You may enjoy reading material that you either read out loud together or read separately and discuss.

If either of you needs a break from constant togetherness, take responsibility for that. Let each other know when you've reached your limit at connecting and you need time alone before you will be ready for more intimacy. You may wish to read a book, jog, walk, or climb a tree. It really doesn't matter as long as you make it clear that you are not rejecting your spouse.

No Distractions

Issues or distractions that get in the way of your connection may already be obvious. For others, you may not be sure of what is likely to pull you apart.

Television is the usual culprit; it causes more trouble in marriages than is imaginable. Most often the husband watches and the wife feels neglected. Talk about the TV issue before the honeymoon. We recommend that the television not even be turned on unless the two of you decide together that you both want to watch. Enjoy watching as a couple, then turn it off. No show, sports event, or news program is worth tension and distance in your relationship. The TV can become a mistress, and most wives do not like sharing their husbands.

Also avoid interruptions from insensitive friends or relatives. You should not be expected to visit with or entertain others on your honeymoon. This is *your* time! Guard it carefully. If you should happen to run into someone you know, decide together how you might handle that. Usually a friendly chat or a stop for coffee is all that is expected. It would be wise to let it be known that you are on your honeymoon. It would probably benefit your privacy to be vague about where you are staying. If someone should drop by to visit you, you have every right to limit his or her stay. You can warmly thank the friend and then let him or her know that this is your time. If directness is difficult for you, tell the friend you have someplace to go and must leave right then. You don't have to say that you are just going for a walk by yourselves. Excuse yourselves and let the friend know you will look forward to seeing him or her sometime after your honeymoon.

Obviously, you as a couple may enjoy time with others. For example, some couples like to return to a family and guest brunch, lunch, or afternoon tea the next day before they leave. If that does not rush your first night, it can be a fun time to connect with those you love, open gifts, and then leave for your more extended honeymoon time.

Rest and Relaxation

It's vital to plan time during your honeymoon for adequate quiet relaxation and rest. This allows for restoration and a more enjoyable time together. It also helps you start your life together in your new home feeling rested.

Activities

Optional activities are a benefit to any honeymoon. These work best if they are flexible rather than scheduled so you can pick and choose what you would like to do and when. Avoid putting money toward an activity so that you feel committed to it. For example, if you buy a golf package, scuba-diving instruction, or a sunset cruise, you will feel obligated to do that activity even though it turns out not to be the best focus for you at that time.

However, if you are an activity-oriented couple, you may prefer to plan your favorite activities into your honeymoon. Hiking, mountain climbing, biking, and camping can be physically draining for some people and not leave much energy to enjoy the new sexual relationship, but others find they need strenuous physical activity to keep their sexual vitality alive.

It is most important that you not plan an activity you love but your partner does not. An afternoon in the hot sun watching your favorite team lose another game may not be your spouse's idea of a great honeymoon. Even if this is your first chance to see a game in person, *forget it!* On the other hand, if you both are rabid fans and you met at a game, this might be an exciting way to spend a day. Work it out, but don't talk him or her into it. You will regret it! The honeymoon should be designed for both people's pleasure and enjoyment.

A man may really get into a sporting event, but totally lose his wife. Or the woman may plan a shopping spree and find herself with an irritable husband. You will have plenty of time during your married lives to engage in the activities of your choice; this is not the time for pursuing individuation.

Tour groups can be a distraction. If your time is controlled by a scheduled tour group for ten days, you will not be free to respond to your own timing needs and desires. You may decide to visit a museum or a scenic or historic site, and that will not take away from your focus on each other. But avoid committing yourselves to anything that is prescheduled. Your honeymoon is one of the few times you may have in life to do what you want to do when you want to do it.

No Surprises

The honeymoon is most likely to be enjoyed by both of you if there are no surprises. If you absolutely do not like to be taken by surprise, make certain your spouse-to-be truly understands how adamant you are about that before you plan the honeymoon. If he or she believes a particular surprise would be an exception and goes ahead against your warning, that can put you in a dilemma. It will be impossible to act like you are delighted when you may feel furious; in response, your partner may be crushed by your reaction.

On the other hand, if you love to be surprised, let your spouse-to-be know that. You may want to bring some little surprises for each other to enhance your romantic responsiveness.

If you don't feel strongly either way about being surprised, be cautious. Avoid major surprises. The risk is too great that you might not get the positive response you expect; your idea may not bring the joy you had hoped it would.

Likewise, avoid any major investment of time or money in something neither of you has ever tried. It would not be wise to plan a fishing trip on a lake in northern Minnesota in August if you have never been to Minnesota in August and have never tried fishing. Nor would it be a good idea to plan your dream sailing trip if you had never sailed. You might get seasick and spend your entire honeymoon feeling nauseous. Similarly, if you are from the prairie and have always wanted a vacation in the mountains, this is not the time to find out if you're prone to altitude sickness. If you have not been out in the sun, be cautious about a tropical island setting; sunburned bodies do not make for a delightful honeymoon.

Establishing Patterns

This is the beginning of your married life, and you will be establishing lifelong patterns of interaction and role responsibilities: Who checks in with the airlines? Who calls the cab? Who checks you in at the hotel? Who handles tipping? Who takes responsibility to correct situations that did not happen as you had planned? Who showers first? Who initiates closeness? Who initiates bedtime? Do you keep the window open or closed? How dark do you have the room for sleeping? Which side of the bed do you sleep on? Who sets the alarm? How close to each other do you sleep? Do you need bathroom privacy? How do you squeeze out and put the cap on the toothpaste? What do you do with used towels or dirty clothes? The list of issues to be addressed could go on forever. For some couples, these decisions seem to happen uneventfully. Others encounter many differences and have a greater need for deliberately developing patterns of responsibility to enhance their relationship and their individual well-being.

Not all patterns will be established on the honeymoon; you will have a lifetime of learning to live together with ease. You can design your honeymoon to be virtually free of any need to determine lifetime patterns, or you may have to address these issues. For example, staying at a cabin and doing your own cooking would be more similar to most couples' ongoing life, while being on a cruise or in a hotel where all services are taken care of would be free of most normal life decisions or pattern-setting. Choose how you would like to use this honeymoon time to benefit you most.

Location

Setting. Privacy is a central criterion in planning your honeymoon. To feel free to express yourselves sexually, you will want to make certain you are not heard by and do not hear your neighbors. That is why bed-and-breakfast inns are not a wise choice—they are usually old, restored homes. The walls are not well insulated for sound, there is space under the door, and the wooden floors and beds usually creak with any movement.

Not only do you want sound protection, you also want privacy from socializing expectations with other people. This is another negative for bed-and-breakfasts as honeymoon sites. Communal mealtimes will take away from your ability to exclusively focus on your relationship and will obligate you to eat at certain preset times.

Cleanliness and decor can be important issues to some individuals. Some people have strong preferences for the stark newness of a modern setting as opposed to a country setting with antiques, handwoven rugs, a rock fireplace, and worn furniture. Some people's moods are affected by the lightness or darkness of their room. Earth tones may make your spirits dip; bright colors may energize you.

The cleanliness of a place would not even be noticed by some people and would ruin the honeymoon for others. If you are wondering what importance these external elements have to two people who love each other deeply and enjoy each other's presence, then you can skip these considerations. Just be certain your spouse feels the same way!

Weather. The weather can affect the setting, the activities, and you. If you don't like rain, do not honeymoon in Seattle in November. If humidity makes you sluggish and leaves you feeling that you do not want to be touched, don't honeymoon in Georgia in July. If you hate cold as much as Joyce does, do not go on a snow skiing vacation. If dry heat bothers you, stay away from the desert city of Palm Springs, California, in August when it is 125 degrees. Wind invigorates some and irritates others; avoid Chicago if you are the latter. No one likes mosquitoes, but if you are bothered more than a little (i.e., if you get huge welts from bites) you will want to make certain you do not choose a location that is swarming with mosquitoes or other insects.

Geography. There is nothing that makes a beach honeymoon better than a mountain honeymoon or a lake honeymoon. You might prefer to honeymoon in the desert or on a lake, at a coast or beach, in the mountains, on the plains, in a city, or on an island. The type of scenery and location is a personal choice.

Travel. How you prefer to travel may affect the location you choose. If you are afraid of flying, that will limit your choices to travel by ground or sea. Some people's ears are severely affected by the change in air pressure when they fly. If that is true for you, you may need to get medication to reduce or eliminate that complication, which often makes people irritable after a flight.

You may have a personal preference or idiosyncrasy that will affect your choice of travel. Some couples love a leisurely driving trip. That would not have worked for us. While vacationing in northern Minnesota for our August honeymoon, Cliff wanted to take Joyce to see the Northshore Drive of Lake Superior, which reminded him of the beautiful evergreens of his British Columbia home. After driving fifteen miles, Cliff noticed that Joyce was asleep. He stopped so we could look at a beautiful scene (and to wake up Joyce), then we drove on. Before long, Joyce was asleep again. After a third stop, Cliff decided to turn back and go to our cabin. We discovered on that trip that Joyce falls asleep almost as soon as a car starts moving. A ten-day driving trip would have been very restful for Joyce and very lonely for Cliff.

Train travel can be fun, free of responsibility, and very relaxing. The bed and privacy situation would not be a great setting in which to spend most of your nights, however. And you might feel too much a part of a "community" because many train travelers enjoy getting acquainted with fellow passengers. But it's also possible to remain anonymous.

Travel by water is high risk unless you are experienced sea travelers. Seasickness definitely deadens a sexual relationship. Cruises can be fun but may also feel too confining within a communal-type situation. Thus, cruises carry many of the negatives of a bed-and-breakfast inn.

How you travel is a matter of personal preference, or your destination may dictate your choice of travel.

RESPONSIBILITIES

Traditionally, the man plans and pays for the honeymoon, but that is not a rule. We believe you will be happiest with your honeymoon if you plan it together. The financial responsibility can be shared or assumed by anyone. It is important that the money spent on the honeymoon is realistic. A glamorous honeymoon that eats up all your financial resources will leave you in a rough situation when you return home, and there's unlikely to be much sympathy from your parents. If you will be sharing income and expenses after the honeymoon, you should decide together how much you can spend without affecting your living arrangements afterward.

What if the man is just not a planner and arranger? Work together. Divide the responsibilities. Together decide which ones each of you does better. Whoever does telephone negotiations better should call to make various reservations. The other one of you may have better organizational skills. This is a great time to learn more about what each of you does well. It is better for the one who is a natural at some task to assume that responsibility. Just make sure the responsibilities basically even out.

TROUBLESHOOTING

Ideally, your thorough preparation will prevent any need for troubleshooting. But be prepared, just in case you have difficulties. Take the telephone numbers of your medical doctor, your premarital counselor, and any other resources you might need. Feel free to give us a quick call at (626) 449-2525 or e-mail us at penners@attglobal.net. If you call, be sure to leave your telephone and room number on our voice message. Sometimes five minutes of correct guidance can make all the difference in the world. If you need to pursue more involved counseling, we can refer you to some professional in your area, or we can arrange for ongoing paid appointments by telephone. For sure, take *Sex 101*!

■ ■ ■

I've heard it doesn't matter where we go for our honeymoon, because we're just going to stay in our room and have sex all the time.

The honeymoon is often a time of sexual and personal adjustment. Whether or not there has been sexual activity before marriage, the stress and excitement of the wedding as well as the awareness of your now being husband and wife can cause you to change.

On your honeymoon, and in your marriage every day thereafter, the "normal" frequency of sex is what the two of you determine is right *for you*. That could be twice per day, twice per week, or twice per month. The key is to negotiate the best balance of your natural sexual desires.

I want our sex to always be exciting and spontaneous. How do you avoid getting into a sexual rut?

In movies and romantic novels, exhilarating sex is spontaneous. The couple's eyes meet across the room, and they are so drawn to each other that they slip away to some corner and make mad, passionate love before they hardly know each other's names. In real life, the more preparation, anticipation, talking, guiding, and scheduling you put into your sexual times with each other, the better they likely will be. If you wait for some mysterious erotic energy to grab you before you have sex, you may not be having sex very often. The most satisfying sexual encounters between you and your spouse will often be the ones you plan for and talk about.

The best way not to get into a rut is to allow quality time for your sex life and to learn to guide each other in the sexual experience. If each of you takes responsibility to listen to each other's needs and desires and communicate them to one another without demand, you won't have to keep trying to figure out what works and then keep doing over and over what worked once. Rote repetition of what worked once is a sure way to get into a rut and diminish the spark of your sexual relationship.

5 PREPARE FOR YOUR FIRST TIME

By reading and sharing this book, you have already begun the process of opening your sexual inner worlds to each other. Whether or not this is your first sexual intercourse experience, there are specific steps you can take to make that first time after your wedding an event that is associated with lasting positive memories. In this chapter we'll discuss those important preparations.

PREPARE YOUR MINDS

Your most influential and positive sex organ is your mind; it controls your body, how you think about sex, how you feel about sex, and how your body responds to sex. What is your mind-set toward sex in marriage? In the following pages we'll discuss five basic attitudes we hope you have already acquired. If these attitudes are not representative of your mind-set about sex and marriage, we hope you will attempt to integrate these into your way of thinking.

Sex Is Good and of God

Sex was God's idea. God created us male and female in His image (Gen. 1:27–28). And when God completed His work of creation, He looked at His work and was pleased. It was good! So our sexuality, our differences and uniqueness as men and women, are part of God's perfect, sinless design for us. Then God instructed men and women how they were to live with one another. He told the man to leave his mother and father and become one with his wife. This was the instruction to consummate their physical relationship—to become one physically, emotionally, and spiritually (Gen. 2:24). This sexual union was part of God's perfect design for mankind.

Sexual Curiosity Is Natural

As human beings grow from infancy to adulthood, it becomes evident that God's design of our sexuality includes a natural pursuit of sexual discovery. Your interest in knowing each other sexually is completely natural. There is no need to feel guilt or shame or embarrassment while exploring one another as a married couple. The freedom to become comfortable and familiar with each other will grow gradually for some. Others will be unashamed of their curiosity about each other right from the start. Be sensitive to your individual needs in that regard, and be sensitive to each other's needs for privacy, as well as for familiarity. As Paul Popenoe wrote in *Preparing for Marriage*:

> The change from the restrictions of the engagement period to the freedom of marriage is, in many cases, made too rapidly. There is a gap which must be bridged over carefully, by a steady process of mutual education and adjustment during the engagement, and by continuing this uninterruptedly after the

wedding. The inherent tendency of all male animals to delight in exhibiting themselves must be repressed, particularly on the wedding night and during the early part of the honeymoon, if a modest and sensitive bride is not to be distressed.[1]

Popenoe's book was originally written in 1938 and was the marriage manual we used in preparation for our marriage. In preparing to write this book, we went back to look at both current and original manuals, and this book continues to amaze us with its relevancy.

Many of the unconsummated marriages we see in sexual therapy started with the bride tensing up on her wedding night when her husband surprised her with his nude body and a full erection.

It would be best to assume your curiosity about each other on the wedding night will begin with the degree of openness you have experienced with each other before marriage. Gradually continue learning to know more about each other as you grow in trust and familiarity after marriage. Eventually, it will be helpful to your sexual relationship to become specifically familiar with each other's genitals and teach each other about the genital touching that is most pleasurable to you.

Sexual Responsiveness Is Inborn

Your bodies confirm the perfect design of God's creative power. Your responsiveness demonstrates the beauty of how your bodies have been set in motion sexually.

Sexual responsiveness is an involuntary response. It is not an action you can *will* or make happen by a mental decision. But it is a response you can *allow* to happen by a positive, sexually assertive attitude.

You can encourage this response in your marriage by honoring the fact that both of you were born as sexually responsive people and that sexual responsiveness is to be fulfilled in marriage. Both of you have the privilege of enjoying one another's body to go after that fulfillment. That will work only if sexual enjoyment is pursued for both of you. It must be kept mutual.

The potential for sexual responsiveness is equal for men and women. Physiologically, men are no more or less sexual than women. Men and women have been designed with equal capacity for sexual pleasure and release.

In our society a prevailing attitude about men and women contradicts this concept of equality and causes a lot of destruction in marriage. It assumes that men are more sexual than women and that men have a need and a right for sexual release whether or not the woman does; thus, according to this attitude, the role of the wife is to sexually please her husband. Sexual pleasure in this view is not something the woman seeks out, but rather is something she provides for her husband. It is her job to increase his feelings of masculinity and control and to let him use her body for his pleasure, but not to expect that for herself. This sense of *duty* for a woman to have sex to keep her husband satisfied and at home doesn't work. The wife who is involved sexually *only* to please her husband without going after sexual enjoyment for herself eventually ends up with a husband who is not pleased. As sex becomes a task rather than a pleasure, she becomes less and less responsive, and sexual encounters become an event she dreads. The husband senses her absence of vitality and becomes anxious about her lack of involvement but often doesn't understand what went wrong. Tension and distance build.

This is not an inevitable scenario, however. Pursue your natural responsiveness with vigor but never at the expense of one another.

Sexual Responsibility Belongs to Each Person

Sexual responsiveness has to do with sexual feelings and desires. In contrast, sexual responsibility has to do with the choices you make about those feelings. It is natural to have sexual feelings toward people of the opposite sex at various times throughout life. It is your responsibility not to pursue those feelings or actions with anyone other than your spouse. Sex is not something that happens to you. You can choose to not act on your sexual feelings toward anyone other than your spouse, and you can choose to be sexual with your spouse even when you are not particularly aware of those desires. You can also choose not to pursue sex with your spouse when he or she would perceive that as a demand or violation.

Sexual responsibility is not only important to practice in pursuing your sexual feelings with the correct partner and in being respectful of that partner; it is also vital to practice in your actual sexual experiences.

A popular mentality about men contradicts this attitude of individual responsibility within a sexual relationship. This mentality assumes that men are more qualified sexual partners than are women. Thus, the man is expected to come to marriage with the ability to tactfully and skillfully lead his innocent bride through the most delightful sexual time of her life. According to this mentality, it is his responsibility to turn her on. If he really loves her, according to this theory, he will automatically sense what she likes and doesn't like. Having this innate ability, he will sensitively woo her to a state of ecstatic arousal and release. Meanwhile, she is the passive receptor of his natural male skills. As one woman expressed it, "He's got to do something to turn me on."

When either the husband or the wife puts this demand on the man, it gets in the way of open communication and mutual enjoyment. Neither of them ends up happy! Even Dr. Popenoe recognized this reality when he wrote in *Preparing for Marriage,* "It is indispensable to the husband's happiness that his wife be a real partner, not a silent and passive instrument."[2] To demand that the husband be responsible for the wife's pleasure will only cause anxiety and frustration. You both need to learn to listen to the desires of your bodies, take responsibility to communicate those desires to each other, and go after them—letting each other know what you would enjoy but never demanding or violating the other.

Assuming responsibility for your sexuality outside of marriage will help prevent unintended sexual encounters from happening. Assuming responsibility for your sexuality within marriage will reduce demand, allow greater freedom, and help protect your marriage from sex with someone other than your spouse.

Mutual Respect Is the Guide for All Sexual Relationships

Mutual respect is essential for the enjoyment of sex in marriage. Never should any activity take away from your closeness with God or be something that is negative for one of you. There are enough ways that you, as a couple, can enjoy ingenuity, zest, and vitality in your sex life without interfering with either of these primary commitments. When a husband and wife respect each other's feelings and desires, they are free to enjoy each other's bodies with mutual abandonment.

If you begin your sexual relationship in marriage by believing and practicing these five principles of biblical teaching on sexuality, your chances for enjoying many years of a free, pleasurable sexual relationship together are very promising.

PREPARE YOUR BODIES

You are going to share your bodies most intimately. To feel most relaxed and open with each other, it is important that your bodies are ready for this experience. If it will be the first time for either or both of you to have sexual intercourse, if it will be the first time for you to have sexual intercourse with each other, or if it will be the first time in a long time, the following preparations will make this a special event.

The Woman's Preparations

Get a recommendation for a gynecologist, medical practitioner, or nurse practitioner who is known to be thorough yet sensitive in examining and guiding women in preparing for marriage. Ask the examining clinician to inform you very specifically of the condition of your genitals and your readiness for sexual intercourse. You may ask about the condition of both your hymen and your vaginal muscle. If either seems tight, you may need to ask for graduated vaginal dilators. Never agree to surgery for relieving tightness unless that treatment is validated by at least two other clinicians.

Be prepared to discuss contraceptive measures. Write out your thoughts and questions after reading chapter 6. If you plan to use a hormonal contraceptive, get started on the hormone of your choice at least two months before your wedding so your body has time to adjust. If you have complications or serious side effects, that will give you time to change to a hormone that interacts differently with your body. When you have the required blood tests for getting your marriage license, ask to be tested for AIDS, herpes simplex II, genital warts, and any other sexually transmitted diseases (STDs) your clinician would recommend. It would also be good to make sure you don't have a yeast infection. If the physician is willing, we would recommend getting a prescription for an antibiotic to treat "honeymoon cystitis," should you get it. Honeymoon cystitis is an infection of the bladder that is common because of the sudden frequent sexual activity. Germs can easily travel into the urinary tract and cause a bladder infection that can be very painful. The pain is usually relieved relatively quickly after appropriate medications are taken.

Regularly exercising the PC (pubococcygeus) muscle of the vagina will enhance sexual sensitivity. Begin by identifying the sensation of tightening and relaxing this muscle. While sitting on the toilet to urinate, spread your legs apart. Start urination. Then stop urination for three seconds. Repeat this several times before you are finished emptying your bladder. If you have difficulty stopping urination, you need to work on tightening the PC muscle. If you have difficulty restarting urination, you need to work on voluntarily relaxing the PC muscle. If you can do both easily, you only need to tighten and relax the muscle twenty-five times per day to keep it in good condition.

You might connect your PC muscle exercise with some regular daily activity, so that activity is a reminder to you. For example, you could do five contractions of the muscle every time the telephone rings. If either tightening or relaxing the PC muscle is difficult for you, follow the instructions below.

1. Gradually tighten the PC muscle tighter and tighter to the count of four. Then hold the muscle as tight as you can while you again count to four. Now gradually relax the muscle, letting go of the tension a little at a time as you count to four. Do ten to twenty repetitions of this exercise one to four times per day.

2. Start to tighten your vagina by thinking of bringing your labia (lips) closer together, like closing an elevator door. Imagine that your vagina is an elevator. You start to tighten at the ground floor. Bring the muscles up from floor to floor, tightening and holding at each floor. Keep your breathing even and relaxed. Do not hold your breath. Continue until you get to the fifth floor. Then go down, relaxing the tension of the muscle one floor at a time. When you get to the bottom, bear down as though you are opening the elevator door (the vagina) and letting something out. Do ten to twenty repetitions of this exercise one to four times per day.

3. Rapidly tighten and relax the PC muscle at the opening of the vagina in almost a flickering or fluttering movement. Do ten to twenty repetitions of this exercise one to four times per day.

In the months before your wedding night, stretch the opening of your vagina every time you bathe or shower. Relaxing in warm water will help you relax your vaginal muscle so you can insert the dilator or your clean fingers. Begin with inserting one finger or a dilator the size of a tampon applicator. If you have difficulty inserting something that size, you can try a cotton-tipped applicator with a lubricant on it. Gradually increase the size of the object you insert to stretch the opening of your vagina until you are able to insert three fingers and stretch them apart or insert the largest dilator. The circumference of an average erect penis is about four and a half to five and a half inches. When you insert the dilator, leave it in the vagina for about twenty minutes per day. The more faithful you are in preparing your vagina for entry, the more comfortable that initial experience will be. Since your vaginal muscle has either never been used for sexual intercourse before or it has been a long time since it has been used, you must think of preparing it for this special event as an athlete would prepare for an athletic event.

Groom your body especially carefully as the time for the wedding gets close. Different cultures and ethnic groups have standards of what is expected bodily preparation. In many Western cultures, the woman is expected to have smooth legs and underarms that have been freshly shaved, epilated, or waxed. If you have concern about other body hair, like above the lip, on the abdomen, or along the bikini line, those may be permanently removed by electrolysis. That must be done long before the wedding date since it is an expensive, tedious process that requires healing afterward. The other hair-removal methods can work just fine if you cannot invest money or time in electrolysis. The primary goal is for both you and your husband to feel good about your body.

The Man's Preparation

Just as the woman should make certain her body is healthy, free from infection, and ready for sexual intercourse, so should the man. It is wise to have a complete physical examination by a medical doctor. If you have any concerns related to your genitals, these can be dealt with at the time of your examination. The privacy of the physician's office is the place to address any questions. If your concerns or questions are minimized by the physician, that is a sign of the physician's inadequacy, not that you asked an inappropriate question. Find another doctor. When you get your blood tested for your marriage license requirements, get tested for AIDS, genital warts, herpes simplex II, and any other sexually transmitted diseases that might be of concern. Testing for sexually transmitted diseases is a gift of trust you give each other. That is true whether or not you have been sexually active previously.

Whatever your practice of masturbation or your past sexual experience has been, you would do yourself and your new wife a big favor if you practiced, through self-stimulation, learning to extend ejaculation. It is important that no self-stimulation be practiced in association with pornography or other addictions.

You can learn ejaculatory control by focusing on and savoring the pleasurable sensations, becoming aware of the warning signs that you are nearing ejaculation, stopping and starting stimulation, and/or squeezing the coronal ridge of the penis. Stimulation must be stopped or the squeeze applied long before you notice you are approaching the point of no return when you are about to ejaculate. Another important ingredient to learning to delay ejaculation is to rest or allow the intensity of the arousal to dissipate while you stop stimulation or apply the squeeze. Then resume stimulation. For more information refer to chapter 16 in our book *Restoring the Pleasure*, Helen Singer Kaplan's book *P.E.: How to Overcome Premature Ejaculation*,[3] or Michael E. Metz and Barry McCarthy's book *Coping with Premature Ejaculation: How to Overcome PE, Please Your Partner, & Have Great Sex*.[4]

Stimulating yourself to ejaculation within twenty-four hours before your wedding night will also be of great benefit to both you and your bride because you will likely be more excited and fatigued than usual and more apt to ejaculate quickly. This can be disappointing to both of you. A recent ejaculation will increase the time of pleasure and enjoyment for this first, memorable, married sexual experience.

Preparations to Do Together

Take time to talk about and decide which contraceptive method the two of you would like to use. The next chapter provides information to help you with this decision. Determine which method has the most likelihood of success and is the most desirable for both of you. Once you have made your decision, obtain all of the necessary supplies you will need to effectively practice this method. Then familiarize yourselves with the process you have chosen.

If you will be using condoms, the man should practice applying the spermicide and the condom. If the diaphragm, cervical cap, sponge, or vaginal condom is your choice, the woman should practice inserting the device until it can be done with ease. If you are following a "natural" family-planning program, you should both be aware of where the woman will be in her cycle at the time of your wedding and honeymoon. Since the excitement surrounding the wedding can disrupt a woman's usual cycle, it might be wise to use an additional contraceptive for your wedding night and honeymoon. Or you might purchase and use an ovulation test kit. That would be an additional expense, but a worthwhile one.

Whatever your method of contraception, it is important that you are comfortable with it and can safely and efficiently use it so you avoid frustration—and an unplanned pregnancy.

Once you have settled on your method of contraception, choose and purchase a lubricant. Since a woman lubricates vaginally early in a sexual experience, a time of long extended love play will require a lubricant. Whether or not you think you will need a lubricant, we recommend that all newly married couples automatically use one and that all couples have a lubricant available. Using a lubricant is not a sign of failure. Rather, to use a lubricant reduces demand and enhances pleasure because you do not have to pay attention to whether or when lubrication is occurring.

If you have chosen to use a rubber (latex) barrier contraceptive method—such as condoms, diaphragms, or cervical caps—you should not use a lubricant that is oil- or petroleum-based. Oil and petroleum decrease the effectiveness of rubber (latex). Thus, you should not use Vaseline or other petroleum jellies, natural oils, mineral oil, butter, grease-based sexual lubricants, or some vaginal creams. You can use aloe, water, saliva, glycerin, and contraceptive foams, creams, and gels; commercial sexual lubricants include Probe, Astroglide, PrePair, Lubrin, Transi-Lube, Aqua-Lube, Condom-Mate, Duragel, and others; and water-based lubricants such as K-Y Jelly or Lubrafax. The water-based lubricants dry more quickly than others on the list, so they are not quite as desirable.

The more carefully you have prepared your bodies for one another and the better prepared you are, the more positive your first sexual experience together will be. So take time to prepare carefully, and deliberately try to anticipate your every need and desire.

Prepare Your Spirits and Souls

You will not just be joining your bodies; you will be joining all of who you are. Throughout the busy times of planning for and enjoying the events connected with your wedding, you will need to carve out time for yourselves, individually and together. Make certain you take time to keep your spirits and souls nurtured. If you come to the wedding and honeymoon totally depleted, you will have nothing to give and may even have difficulty receiving. Even if you take just fifteen minutes each day to read, reflect, and pray, you will give yourself a great gift to prepare your inner spirits for each other. To keep your spirits connected, you might share a similar daily or weekly time together. Also, frequent walks and talks can help relieve stress and keep you connected.

Make a detailed time plan for the week of the wedding. Be realistic about allotting enough time for the required tasks; even when you think you've designated enough time, allow more.

Plan to do very few tasks yourself. Be bold; ask friends and family members to help. Make task lists. Block out time each day for a nap. It will be important to spend time with family and friends who are visiting from out of town, so try to arrange relaxed settings where these guests can gather and enjoy time with you, but keep these times limited.

The day of the wedding is most critical. Plan your day so that you can sleep in as long as your body will allow you (unless you have a morning wedding). The rest of the day should include as much rest and pampering as time allows. You may want to get ready for the ceremony with the help of your wedding attendants or just your family or by yourself. If you are a person who is energized by being with people, you probably will want others around. If you get fatigued and need to restore your energy by being alone for a while, plan some rejuvenation time into the day's schedule.

■ ■ ■

Are you at risk for contracting an STD if you have never had sexual intercourse?

If neither you nor your spouse have had genital-to-genital, oral-to-genital, or genital-to-anal contact, you are not at risk of contracting most STDs. Sometimes an individual who has not been sexually active can carry the virus that causes genital warts. It may remain dormant for years and become activated during sexual intercourse. Authorities are not certain how the person's body acquired the virus in the first place. It might have been through sharing used swimming suits or public swimming pools. The oral herpes simplex I virus may have been transferred to the genitals through oral-genital stimulation. We recommend that you both be tested for STDs whether or not you have engaged in behaviors that transmit them. It will take care of any doubts and build trust that the two of you are starting clean with each other.

If I was tested for AIDS six months after my last sexual contact, do I need to be tested again?

Yes, you do. The virus causing AIDS may not show up on a blood test until after six months, so you need to keep getting tested every six months until the wedding. Usually you will be considered safe after a year, but new information is continually being made available on the reliability of AIDS testing, so call an AIDS testing service for the current information.

How do I deal with the memories of past sexual partners, positive and negative? What can I (or we) do now to minimize the negative effects my past may have on our marriage?

This is a difficult, yet common, struggle for many couples entering marriage today. We believe the Bible's teaching that sex is for marriage was designed to prevent this very dilemma. The conditions of married sex are different from sex outside of a committed relationship. Unmarried sex is often associated with risk, guilt, winning, keeping, conquering, rebelling, and/or deceiving. If your previous sex was connected with any of these conditions, you will need to "undo" that past so it won't negatively affect your sex life in your marriage. Memories of past sexual partners easily move into the marriage bed with you. They may show up in your marriage as comparisons, self-doubt, distrust, dissatisfaction, or fear.

How you deal with your fiancé is important. It is important to tell him or her that your past still affects you and that you want to be free of it and get it out of the way of your current relationship. Do not share details of that past; otherwise the memories will also haunt your fiancé. Share how it affects you, what you have done about it, and how you would like to work together to minimize or eliminate its effects on your marriage.

Listen to, reflect, and care about your fiancé's feelings about your past. It will be easy for you to get defensive if his or her reaction is one of hurt, anger, or distrust. The more you understand that your fiancé's reactions are most natural, the sooner they will decrease.

Finally, together make a plan for dealing with this past within your marriage. Start as if your married sexual relationship is the first experience for both of you. Learn about each other as unique sexual beings totally different from those past partners. Do not start sexually at the place you left off. Start as a new learner. Let your spouse teach you about himself or herself. When that past sneaks in, have a plan to signal each other and distract from those thoughts, feelings, or comparisons and focus more diligently on each other. Continually affirm your love and commitment to each other by your words and your actions. You will need to be more deliberate about this than someone without past sexual partners.

We have decided to wait for marriage to consummate our sexual relationship. That used to be a struggle for us, but it no longer is. Could we have shut off our feelings for each other?

It certainly sounds as if that may be what happened. When we teach premarital classes, we always caution that if a premarital couple has decided not to be sexually active before marriage and it is not a struggle for them, they better get some help. God has designed us to desire sexual intimacy with the person we love and commit ourselves to. That is our responsiveness. We are given the responsibility to manage that drive so we do not violate ourselves, our partner, or our relationship with God. Therefore, sexual activity should be controlled by the decisions we make and the conditions we put ourselves into, not by turning off our desire for that intimacy.

Since the two of you seem to have already turned off your "pilot lights," it is time to relight those desires. Saying "I do" will not turn the switch back on. Between now and your wedding, reengage in times of passionate kissing that go no farther than that. If you sense an urge for more, affirm those good feelings by telling each other about them, but stick to just kissing. As desire builds, allow yourselves more bodily contact, but always after deciding upon very clear behavioral boundaries that will keep with your desires to wait for marriage. Don't allow your actions to go farther than what you have decided upon. Affirm your desires, but control the level of your sexual involvement by the settings you allow yourselves to be in and the physical behaviors you allow yourselves to engage in.

6 FAMILY-PLANNING OPTIONS

Preparation for your wedding night—and for your life as husband and wife—will include consideration of whether you want to use contraceptives and if so, what method is best for both of you. Many couples assume the responsibility to plan the number of children they hope to have and when they hope to have them. Family planning is the process of setting up that program for your reproductive life. It is thinking, praying, and talking with each other about this decision. Whenever a couple decides not to allow the wife to get pregnant any time that would happen naturally, they have chosen to control conception.

As you come to grips with the religious and moral issues of contraception, you will work through those issues together. It is best if the family-planning decisions are settled before marriage. Ask yourselves, "How does our reproductive plan fit with our religious beliefs? Would we like to have children? How old would we like to be when we have children? How would we feel if we couldn't have children? How would we feel if we got pregnant without planning for it?"

Each of you comes to the marriage with attitudes regarding

childbearing that will affect your feelings about using contraception. These attitudes need to be cleared with each other. One spouse may be totally against using contraception and the other not ready to allow babies to arrive at random. Agreement concerning your attitudes and feelings about contraception is vital to family planning—and to your marriage.

MAKING THE CHOICE

Contraception prevents the man's sperm from uniting with the egg cell from the woman. Note that contraception is used to prevent pregnancy, not to interrupt it once conception has taken place. That is an important moral and religious distinction. We are not talking about taking life; we are talking about preventing a new life from beginning.

There is no perfect method of contraception. What works well for one couple may not be suitable for another. All methods currently practiced have both advantages and disadvantages. The method you choose will be as effective as you are in using it.

Today a variety of reliable methods are available. Choosing a proper contraceptive method is a serious matter. It is not the woman's decision. It is a decision to be made by both spouses with thought and care. In choosing a contraceptive, four issues need to be considered: safety, effectiveness, convenience, and personal preference.

Remember, if you are not going to faithfully use the method you choose, it will not be effective even if it is, by general definition, safe, effective, and convenient. Your personal preference may depend on how a method will interfere with your sexual relations. That is why this issue needs to be discussed by the two of you.

NONMETHODS

Abstinence

Refraining totally from sexual intercourse is 100 percent effective, but is not appropriate for marriage. We believe abstinence is the method of choice before marriage but is clearly against biblical teaching after marriage. First Corinthians 7:3–5 says we are not to withhold ourselves from one another except by agreement for a season of prayer, and then we're to come together again quickly lest we be tempted. Nowhere does the Bible state that we should abstain from sex to prevent pregnancy.

Withdrawal

Having intercourse (entry of the penis into the vagina) but removing the penis from the vagina before the man ejaculates (releases seminal fluid containing sperm) is frequently practiced as an attempt to prevent conception. It is *not* a method of contraception, however, and it has many disadvantages. First, it can be emotionally and physically upsetting. Two people have united themselves intensely; then (and at the height of openness and vulnerability) they pull apart. Second, many men do not have complete control over when they ejaculate, so accidents are almost inevitable. Third, and of utmost importance, seminal fluid containing sperm is released *before* ejaculation. Thus, withdrawal is not effective.

Douching

Using some means to flush the seminal fluid containing sperm out of the vagina has been attempted for ages, but this practice is neither effective nor safe. Those tenacious little sperm are fast and determined; they get into the uterus and go looking for the egg in the fallopian tube long before the woman can get to her douche bag and douching solution! Douching is *not* a method of contraception even though it is thought to be.

BARRIER METHODS

Barrier methods of contraception prevent the sperm from meeting the egg. Barrier contraceptives include condoms for men and for women, the sponge, diaphragms, cervical caps, and spermicides.

Male Condom

A condom is commonly referred to as a rubber, prophylactic, safety, or sheath. It is a latex polyurethane, or animal-membrane device shaped like the finger of a glove that is placed over the erect penis before entry into the vagina.

Reasons for the condom's popularity are their inexpensiveness, their advantage of being easy to purchase without a physician's prescription, and the fact that they require the man's involvement and prevent a woman's allergic reaction to the man's sperm. Except for the occasional allergic reaction to latex, there are no side effects from the use of condoms, so they are safe.

Condoms' effectiveness depends on how they are used. The failure rate as reported by the Food and Drug Administration in August of 2002 is 11 percent.[1] This means that 11 out of 100 couples using condoms perfectly for one year got pregnant. To use condoms successfully, you must be certain the condom is new and free of holes or tears, and follow the detailed instructions for application and withdrawal.

Condoms will be inconvenient; love play must be interrupted to put them on, and the man must keep an erection until he withdraws from the vagina. That can cause considerable anxiety for some men and interfere with their sexual response. Condoms also interfere with some men's pleasure by reducing sensitivity. For others, it is just a nuisance. Repeated experience with putting on condoms as part of the love play can reduce the inconvenience and enhance their use.

Female Condom

This is a polyurethane pouch, or sheath, that lines the inside of the vagina. A flexible ring on each end holds the condom in place. The inside ring is used for insertion and as an internal anchor. The outer ring remains outside the vagina after insertion and covers part of the perineum providing protection to the labia and the base of the penis during intercourse.

The Food and Drug Administration reports a 21 percent failure rate in the first year with typical use.[2] Some women experience irritation and allergic reactions, but the likelihood is reduced since it is not latex and no spermicide is used with the female condom.

The Sponge

The vaginal contraceptive sponge is a two-inch-wide, round, soft, pillow-shaped polyurethane sponge permeated with spermicide (one gram of nonoxynol-9). However, the sponge is not currently marketed.

The Diaphragm

This barrier method has been used effectively for well over one hundred years. The vaginal diaphragm is a dome-shaped rubber with a flexible rim that covers the cervix so that sperm cannot reach the uterus. A spermicidal jelly or cream must be used with a diaphragm to ensure effectiveness since the diaphragm itself cannot prevent all sperm from reaching the cervix.

With typical use, the diaphragm is 83 percent effective in preventing pregnancy. That means seventeen out of one hundred women during the first year of using the diaphragm with spermicide get pregnant. Medications for vaginal yeast infections may decrease effectiveness.[3]

One advantage of the diaphragm is that it has no side effects. Also, it is usually inserted before intercourse and must be left in place for at least six hours after intercourse. The diaphragm must be prescribed and fitted by a physician. The fit should be checked after pregnancy, pelvic surgery, or a weight change of ten pounds or more. The position of the diaphragm should be checked every time you have intercourse.

Cervical Cap

The cap is similar to the diaphragm in function and effectiveness. It is a soft rubber cup with a round rim that fits over the cervix. Just like the diaphragm, the cap needs to be fitted by a professional on a healthy cervix. It comes in four sizes.

The cap has about the same effectiveness as the diaphragm for women who have never been pregnant, but it has a higher failure rate than the diaphragm for women who have been pregnant at least once.[4]

Vaginal Spermicides

Spermicidal creams, jellies, film, foam, suppositories, and tablets inserted into the vagina contain both a carrier and a chemical. The chemical nonoxynol-9 kills the sperm. Spermicidals must be inserted at a designated time before intercourse, depending on the type of spermicide used. The effectiveness of most spermicides lasts an hour. Read the directions of the product you are planning to use to determine when effectiveness begins and how long it lasts.

Studies have shown varying failure rates. The Food and Drug Administration reported that anywhere from 20 to 50 out of 100 women get pregnant using only a spermicide.[5]

Intrauterine Device

The intrauterine device (IUD) is inserted into the uterus by a health professional. The devices have been made of various shapes and materials, including silver, copper, and plastic. A string is attached to the device to allow the woman to check that the IUD is still in place and to allow the physician to remove it. In the 1970s, 10 percent of contraception use in the United States was by the IUD. Today that use is less than 2 percent, and the majority of users are in their thirties and forties. The Centers for Disease Control reports that today's IUDs are highly effective and safe for long-term contraceptive use for women with a low risk of sexually transmitted diseases (STDs).[6]

What about effectiveness? The IUD is considered highly effective. However, the skill of the medical person who inserts the IUD and the woman's checking to make sure it is still in place are essential to its effectiveness. Fewer than 1 percent of women who use the IUD get pregnant.[7]

Convenience is the IUD's biggest advantage. A physician can insert it at any time, even ten minutes after delivering a baby. It can remain in place for ten years; thus, it does not require insertion and removal by the user. Nor does the woman have to remember to take a pill.

How does the IUD prevent pregnancy? For some time, the belief was that the IUD caused abortion by expelling the fertilized egg. This theory is currently in doubt because of a study that collected released eggs from women using the IUD and from women using no form of contraception. Half of the eggs from the women not using contraception had been fertilized and expelled, while none of the eggs from the IUD users showed signs of fertilization.[8] Mirena, the IUD containing a progestin commonly used in birth control pills, works by making the cervical mucus thick and tacky so the sperm become immobilized and cannot enter the uterus.

HORMONAL PREGNANCY PREVENTION

Various forms of hormonal contraception have been researched and debated before and since the approval of "the pill" by the FDA in 1960. Their convenience and effectiveness make them highly desirable.

The Pill

The pill is a combination of synthetic estrogen and progesterone hormones that, when taken by the woman, shuts off the release of eggs so she no longer ovulates. It also inhibits other processes of impregnation. If the pill is started or resumed on the first through the fifth day of the cycle, day one being the first day of any menstrual spotting or bleeding, inhibition of ovulation is virtually assured.

When the pill is taken consistently, it has an effectiveness of 99.7 to 100 percent. When taken at the same time every day as directed and when extra precautions are used when you have diarrhea or vomiting or are taking certain drugs that may interfere with the pill's effectiveness, only one out of one thousand women (0.1 percent) will get pregnant during the first year of use.[9] Most women get pregnant because they stop the pill to validate whether they are having side effects from it. But when they stop the pill, they fail to use other effective contraception. If you want to test the pill's effect on you by going off of it for a while, have other contraception planned and ready to use before you stop.

The ratio and amount of the chemical activity of progesterone, estrogen, and androgen vary with the various types and brands of pills. Each woman's body has to be evaluated to determine which pill will be most effective with the fewest side effects. Unfortunately, some women try one pill, have side effects, and decide this method is not for them. Instead, they may need to change to a lower-level dosage or a pill that has a different proportion of estrogen, progesterone, or androgen.

Managing Contraceptive Pill Patients by Richard P. Dickey can be ordered from Essential Medical Information Systems, Inc., P.O. Box 820062, Dallas, Texas 75382-0062. You may also contact them at 1-800-225-0694 or by going to www.emispub.com. If you are going to use the pill, we recommend that you order this book to help you choose the correct pill for you and to guide you in using it most effectively. As Dr. Dickey says, "I have placed a major emphasis on two indisputable points: 1) patients are different in their responses to OCs [oral contraceptives], and 2) OCs are also different in their steroid contents and, therefore, in the reactions they elicit in patients."[10]

You should be aware that certain medications will interfere with the effectiveness of the pill. Some antibiotics, antifungals, sedatives and hypnotics, anticonvulsants, cholesterol-lowering agents, and other substances may interfere with the pill's ability to prevent pregnancy. This was demonstrated when a granny-to-be wrote a well-known advice columnist saying that her son and daughter-in-law were about to have their first baby. She said the pregnancy was due to the daughter-in-law's ear infection that was treated with antibiotics while she was trusting the pill for pregnancy prevention. If you are on the pill, check with your physician and consult Dr. Dickey's *Managing Contraceptive Pill Patients* before taking any medication. Ask how it interacts with and changes the effectiveness of your hormonal contraceptive.

Benefits. There are other benefits from the pill besides contraception. Premenstrual tension lessons for some women, menstrual cramps may decrease, the duration and amount of blood loss may be reduced, and the time of menstruation becomes totally predictable. Sometimes acne declines, there is less susceptibility to pelvic inflammatory disease, and the risk of ovarian and endometrial cancer is reduced by 40 to 50 percent. The chance of breast cysts and noncancerous breast tumors is lessened by 50 to 75 percent, endometriosis and rheumatoid arthritis are reduced by 50 percent, growth of excessive body hair often diminishes because the OC suppresses androgen activity, and ovarian cysts are reduced by 65 percent.[11]

The pill can also affect a woman's sexuality; about-equal numbers of women report an increase or decrease in sexual desire. Pills with high progesterone activity are likely to suppress desire; pills with high androgen activity encourage desire. Some women find the physical changes with their periods and the reduction of acne enhance their sexual desire and body image. Many women using oral contraceptives do not experience any significant change in sexual behavior, sexual interest, or sexual enjoyment.

Risks Versus Benefits. For women in the high-risk categories, the risks outweigh the benefits, but for the majority of women who are of childbearing age and do not want to get pregnant, the benefits typically outweigh the risks if you meet the following criteria:

- You are a woman in your twenties or thirties.
- You do not weigh more than one-third above your ideal weight.
- You do not smoke.
- You do not have high blood pressure.
- You are not an insulin-controlled diabetic, do not have an elevated cholesterol level or a high LDL/HDL cholesterol ratio, and have not had any female in your extended family develop diabetes or have a heart attack before age fifty.
- You do not have a history of liver, heart, or vascular disease.
- You are not susceptible to blood clotting.

Maximizing Effectiveness. To get the highest effectiveness in pregnancy prevention from oral contraceptives, follow these instructions summarized from *Contraceptive Technology:*[12]

1. Take the pill at the same time every day. Associate taking your pill with something else you do at the same time each day, such as brushing your teeth.

2. Choose a backup method of contraception to use—
   a. During your first month of using the pill for protection
   b. In case you run out of pills
   c. In case you forget to take your pills
   d. If you have to discontinue the pill because of serious side effects

e. If you need protection from sexually transmitted diseases

f. If you have repeated bleeding between cycles

g. If you have to take antibiotics or other medications that interfere with the pill's effectiveness

3. Start your pills according to your physician's instructions and take one pill a day until you finish the pack. If you have a twenty-eight-day pack, begin a new pack immediately. If you are using a twenty-one-day pack, start your new pack one week after you stopped the last pack.

4. Check your pack of birth control pills each morning to make sure you took your pill the day before.

5. If you forget to take your birth control pill or you start your pack late, follow the instructions below:

If you miss one pill, take that tablet as soon as you remember it. Take your next tablet at the regular time. You probably will not get pregnant but just to be sure, you may want to use a backup method for seven days after the missed pill.

If you miss two pills in a row, then take two tablets as soon as you remember and take two tablets the next day. Then return to your regular schedule but use a backup method of birth control for seven days after two missed tablets.

If you miss three pills in a row you will probably begin your period. Whether or not you are menstruating throw away the rest of your pack and begin your next pack as you did when you first started the method. For example, if you are a Sunday starter begin your next pack on Sunday. If you started on any other day, you may simply start your next pack immediately. Use a backup method of birth control until you have been back on pills for seven days.

If the only pills you miss are from the fourth week of a twenty-eight-day pill pack, simply throw away the missed pills. Then continue taking pills from your current package of pills on schedule. The pills in this fourth week do not contain hormones. So missing these pills does not increase your risk for pregnancy at all.[13]

6. "If you have diarrhea or vomiting, use your backup method of birth control until your next period."[14]

7. If you do not have a menstrual period when expected while taking oral contraceptives consult your physician.

8. Read and follow the instructions on the pill package insert.

Injection

Depo-Provera is a deep injection of progestins given every three months to inhibit ovulation. It has the advantages of not being absorbed and processed through the liver and giving moderately long protection. It is not quite as effective in preventing pregnancy as the combined pill, and its contraceptive effects may take six months to reverse.

Patch

Ortho Evra, a skin patch, is worn on the lower abdomen, buttocks, or upper body. It releases both progestin and estrogen directly into the bloodstream. A new patch is applied once a week for three weeks. The patch is not worn during the fourth week so the woman has a menstrual period. The patch has a 1 percent failure rate but appears to be less effective with women over 198 pounds.

Vaginal Contraceptive Ring

The NuvaRing is a flexible ring that is about two inches in diameter. When it is inserted into the vagina, it releases the hormones progestin and estrogen. It is inserted by the woman and remains in place for three weeks. She does not wear the ring during the fourth week and has her menstrual period. The failure rate is 1 percent.[15]

Hormonal methods of contraception are constantly being researched. So new products and current information regarding their effectiveness, risks, and benefits are continually becoming available. Keep yourself informed so your choice is based on fact rather than fear.

NATURAL METHODS

More and more couples today are considering "natural" methods of family planning because they fear the potential risks and side effects of contraceptives. These methods are based on the principle of avoiding sexual intercourse during the woman's fertile phase of the menstrual cycle. "Rhythm," or "Billings," method may be terms you've used to describe natural family planning. We cannot provide enough information here to train you to effectively practice natural family planning, but you can access information about the Billings-ovulation method on the Web at www.billings-ovulation-method.org. Or try *The Ovulation Method: Natural Family Planning* by John J. Billings, which details every dimension of planning pregnancies without using contraceptives or sterilization.[16]

For disciplined, determined, well-trained couples, natural family planning has been successful and enjoyable. One of the benefits is increased awareness of your hormonal cycle. You can enhance your sexual relations by exploring total-body pleasure without intercourse during your fertile or questionable days.

Surgical Sterilization

The opposite extreme of natural family planning is sterilization, a final form of contraception. It ends one's capacity to reproduce.

Male vasectomy is the simplest and safest form of surgical sterilization; this procedure prevents the live sperm from reaching the penis. The sperm normally travel from the testes, where they are produced, through the vas deferens, a tube that leads through the prostate gland to the urethra. During a vasectomy, a small portion of the vas deferens is removed and the cut ends are tied off and sometimes cauterized. This procedure interrupts the sperm's journey so sperm will not be released when a man ejaculates during a sexual experience. He will still produce seminal fluid since some of that is produced in the portion of the duct system above the cut.

One caution: After a vasectomy, a man may have to ejaculate twenty-five times or more before all live sperm are cleared from the duct system above the cut. Several seminal fluid specimens should be taken to the laboratory for confirmation that the sterilization process is complete.

For the woman, sterilization is referred to as tubal ligation. The woman's fallopian tubes are blocked so the egg and sperm cannot meet. It is a one-time surgical procedure through a small incision in the abdominal wall or through the vagina or the uterus. Many times hospitalization is not necessary.

When tubal methods fail, which is less than 1 percent of the time, it is because the procedure itself failed due to the surgeon's misjudgment; there are some other surgical risks involved as well.

Neither male nor female sterilization changes the person's sexuality in any way. The woman will still produce eggs, and the man will still produce sperm. These eggs and sperm disintegrate and are absorbed. The woman continues to menstruate. The man does not usually notice a change in his ejaculation. Hormonal production remains normal for both. Sexual responsiveness and behavior are unaffected except for feeling greater freedom and not having to use contraceptives.

Family planning is a very personal matter. Personal feelings, as well as the technical facts, are important parts of your choice of planned conception. Talk openly with each other about this issue and take responsibility for your sexuality with a focus on the long-term benefits. Choosing a family planning method is not an easy decision because no method is perfect in both effectiveness and safety. Yet everything has risk, including life itself. Remember that no known contraceptive has a death rate as high as pregnancy—and the death rate from pregnancy is very low.

■ ■ ■

Since it is the woman who gets pregnant, shouldn't she take responsibility for birth control?

It is certainly true that the woman carries the baby and so needs to feel secure about the method of birth control used. But the responsibility for choosing a particular method needs to be a joint one because it will affect both the husband and the wife. The woman can easily feel alone in making this decision, so husband, don't desert your wife on this one.

Should we avoid having sex during menstruation and pregnancy?

Not necessarily. Some women will have their highest interest and peak responsiveness during menstruation or pregnancy, possibly because they are not afraid of getting pregnant. You must discover for yourselves what is most comfortable and what brings the most enjoyment for both of you.

7 YOUR WEDDING NIGHT

It is in the sexual experience that we have the possibility of reaching the highest peaks of ecstasy. Because of the powerful potential of sex, the wedding night is an anniversary event, the significant turning point in every couple's relationship. You now are each other's. You have a whole life of togetherness to look forward to. What happens between the two of you that night will be imprinted on your memory forever. In those moments all by yourselves, after the many days of preparation and anticipation, you are free to abandon all previous restrictions. You will no longer have to leave each other and go to your separate living places. You can relinquish all physical boundaries. However the two of you have functioned sexually thus far, this is a first!

What can you do to make your wedding night a special time that leaves you with warm, wonderful feelings? The two of you bring to this night your own unique needs and desires. Your wedding, the reception, the travel to where you will be staying, and the actual setting of that first night will also affect your time together. Whatever your specific circumstances are, we believe there are some basic criteria to a "successful" wedding night for every bridal couple. We'll share those suggestions in this chapter.

REALISTIC EXPECTATIONS

The planning you've done and the discussions you've had regarding your first time together as a married couple—when it is time to consummate your marriage—will help you set clear expectations. Those realistic discussions are key to your wedding night.

Timing

Allow plenty of time. We recommend you allow at least twelve hours between arrival at the hotel and your departure. The ideal would be between twelve and eighteen hours.

Feelings

Expect a wide range of possible feelings. You may be excited to be alone together, or you may be sad because you are leaving your home and family. You may be eager to enjoy each other's body sexually and may have no sense of reservation about sharing yourself completely and openly, or you may be hesitant and fearful. You may be energized, or you may be exhausted. You may feel like being tender and close, or you may feel intensely erotic. There is no ideal; the only "requirement" is that the two of you let each other know what you feel and accept each other's needs for that night. Success means you connect and enjoy where you are rather than try to measure up to some false expectation of how you *should* feel the first night.

Preparation

Allow for bodily preparation. If it has been a long time since you showered, shaved, and brushed your teeth, taking time to freshen your bodies for your time together will refresh you and increase your desirability to your spouse. Prepare any contraceptive measures you plan to use. Make sure you have all the necessary supplies and are very familiar with their use.

Connection

Allow for emotional and spiritual connection. You may want to talk through the details of the wedding. Perhaps taking some time to reflect on Scripture passages that you or someone else chose for your wedding ceremony will be a time of inviting God into your marriage—whatever works for you. Joyce read our Scripture passage out loud and we prayed together on the way to the hotel, so as not to take time once we got there! Be sure you are connected emotionally and spiritually before proceeding sexually.

Sexual Activity

Allow for pleasure without any goal-oriented demands. Remember lovemaking is just that. It is a time of delighting in your bodies without any need for arousal, orgasm, or intercourse. You may want to prepare your bodies and then just enjoy falling asleep in each other's arms. You may enjoy a time of passionate kissing and fondling and then fall asleep and continue later that night or in the morning when you wake up. Or you may enjoy the pleasure of each other's body and a full sexual experience. Before you move ahead, take plenty of time to enjoy the type of physical connection you engaged in before marriage.

What is most important is that you don't go further than both of you desire. Let the most tired, conservative, or hesitant one set the pace and the boundaries. One spouse's pushing for more than the other desires will be remembered negatively for years to come. The consequences are not worth getting what you want at that moment! Limit sexual activity the first night to what both of you would freely desire.

Success

Define success for your first night so that there is no way you can fail. If your only expectation for your wedding night is that you both enjoy being together without any demands to do more than the most hesitant of you desires, then you will surely succeed and have no regrets. Many first nights are made less than ideal by comparison with some external standard, but if you don't set such a standard, your wedding night can be ideal for you.

Expect to feel many emotions as you experience the realities of fatigue, adjustment to each other, being newly married, the newness of your setting, and for some, the "firsts" of your sexual activity. Recognize that you have the honeymoon and many years following it to get to know each other totally. You will grow in your sexual enjoyment as you become more comfortable communicating clearly exactly what touch and sexual activities you find most exciting.

THE SEXUAL EXPERIENCE

It is not important whether you consummate your marriage (have your first married sexual intercourse) on the wedding night, the next day, or later during your honeymoon. It *is* important that you do not avoid each other. After a while, if you have not had sex and one of you is getting concerned about that, call time-out. Find out what is going on and how you might help.

Whenever you have sex for the first time after your wedding, *go slowly!* So many times, couples who have waited for marriage to have sexual intercourse are so eager (just as we were) that they bypass all the wonderful caressing, kissing, and fondling that were such a vital part of their physical interaction before. Now that they can do the "real thing," couples often forget about caressing, or they think the caressing and kissing are not necessary. But that is what made their bodies so hungry for the real thing; when they skip all that intense connecting, the sexual experience can be very quick and leave both feeling disappointed.

We recommend that you spend at least as much time enjoying the pleasure of each other's body as you would have on any date or time together before marriage. You might begin with your clothes on. As arousal and desire for more builds, gradually take off each other's clothes. Again, let the more hesitant one lead.

We often recommend that married couples begin their sexual times by bathing or showering together. That is a way to relax, connect, and prepare your bodies for each other. If this idea sounds good to both of you, try it.

We would recommend playful genital touching under the

water and plenty of time before and/or after to really be passionate with each other before pursuing direct, erotic stimulation. In or out of the bath, touch, talk, kiss, and explore every inch of one another's body to the degree that you both feel free to do that. Soak in the good feelings of being touched and touching. Have fun as you do. Nibble on each other. Let each other know how much you enjoy the other. As you enjoy yourselves, if anything you do is negative for the other, positively invite a different touch or activity. For example, if a touch is too light and ticklish, ask for a heavier touch. Or if kissing gets too intense or forceful, invite softer lips.

As you become ready for direct genital stimulation, invite that by guiding your partner's hand to your genitals or rubbing your genitals against your partner's body. Explore and learn together what feels good. Do not expect that you will automatically know how to touch each other in the way that feels best. Accept your spouse's guidance as a loving desire to enhance the experience for both of you and take away demand for you to automatically know what feels right to him or her.

Allow the arousal to build in waves, enjoying the genital stimulation and then moving to other parts of the body. You want to keep each other hungry for more touch, not saturated so that you get irritated with the stimulation. This is particularly true for women. Direct clitoral stimulation is often more irritating than it is arousing. Most women prefer a flat hand over the clitoral area or fingers on either side of the clitoris to stroke the shaft rather than the tip of the clitoris. Direct stimulation can quickly, with a slight shift in its intensity or location, change from causing peak arousal to instant pain. That is why it is so important for you, the woman, to signal your husband to let him know what you desire—because there is no other way he can know what you need and know when the stimulation gets too intense. You, the man, would do better to vary the stimulation automatically and keep your wife wanting more. If you, as the woman, want to be stimulated to orgasm before entry and that is not a demand for performance but comes from the level of your arousal, go for it!

Entry should be attempted only at the woman's invitation. It is her body that is being entered; therefore, she should guide the penis into her vagina. When you, the woman, feel ready to allow entry, let your husband know that you desire him. It might be easiest for you to get on top of him while he is on his back. He or you can apply lubricant to his penis and separate your labia (lips) and apply lubricant to the opening of your vagina. Use his penis as a paintbrush over the opening of your vagina and on your clitoris. Poke the penis into your vagina just a little. Tighten and relax your PC muscle as you do. Intentionally relax your vaginal muscle as you guide his penis in. You may need to push against his penis to push through your hymen and vaginal muscle.

If you experience resistance, it is usually because the labia are stuck together, you're pushing at the wrong place (that is, you are not quite at the opening or do not have the penis at quite the right angle to enter the vagina), your hymen is a little tough to break, or your vaginal muscle is not relaxed. The latter is the most likely. Remember you are both new at this; just enjoy the process of trying. Play around with different positions if one doesn't work. Stretch or dilate the vagina and try again. Get a hand mirror and together try to figure out what is happening. Do not keep trying until you are frustrated. Stop while the attempts are fun, get some sleep, and pursue pleasure again when you have time to do so leisurely and are not tired. Don't rush to try entry, but continue to pleasure one another. Play with attempts at entry in the process of enjoying each other. If frustration ensues, seek help.

When the penis actually enters the vagina, you may want to stop, withdraw, celebrate, and try entry again later. Or you may just lie quietly together and enjoy the closeness of this special moment. Then gradually build rhythmic thrusting. Rest every now and then to slow down the process and enjoy every sensation. Engage in kissing, breast stimulation, and clitoral stimulation while you are resting together. When you both decide you are ready to thrust to ejaculation, build the frequency and intensity of the thrusting gradually. Think of trying to enjoy every moment and make it last as long as possible, like licking your favorite ice-cream cone. Resist the urge to thrust or to pursue ejaculation. That will end your time quickly and may be disappointing. If that should happen by mistake, don't get down on yourselves. You have years to learn to extend intercourse. Savor the good feelings of being together and stay connected. If you, the woman, need more stimulation, ask for that. The husband can also offer it.

Spend time talking and cuddling when you finish. Affirm each other. Let each other know what you enjoyed. Share fantasies of other possibilities for sexual play if those ideas don't intimidate. Have tissue, a washcloth, a small towel, or some type of wipes at the bedside to catch the seminal fluid and vaginal secretions after sex. There will be a bit of a mess, but the woman can easily handle that by putting tissue or a washcloth between her legs to catch the secretions as they seep out of her vagina. The man can wipe off his penis as necessary.

It would be quite common, if this is your first sexual experience and you have not been bringing yourselves or each other to orgasm, for the woman not to be orgasmic. When we got married, we didn't really even understand about orgasm so Joyce probably wasn't orgasmic at first, but it wasn't an issue for us. We don't even know whether she was or wasn't. We both loved our times together and remember them, including the wedding night, with great fondness. Now those initial experiences would seem disappointing for us, but they were not disappointing then! And that is appropriate. Our accurate knowledge, lack of unrealistic TV and movie models, and our naïveté prevented us from having any real goals. That was a perfect start for our sexual life together. You, too, need not be disappointed if the orgasmic reflex doesn't happen for you initially. If you are allowing arousal, enjoy that and let it build and extend. Eventually, the reflex of orgasm is likely to get triggered, especially if you are active and uninhibited. If you feel frustrated or feel like crying because you have not had release, recognize that as one way your body may be letting down and releasing the tension buildup of the sexual arousal in your body. Hold each other and share the crying. Do not take it as a sign

of failure and avoid each other. Bring that release into your connected feelings.

■ ■ ■

How important is it for both of us to have clean hands and bodies to protect the other from developing irritations or infections?

It is very important to be clean. Nails should be filed and
smooth, hands should be freshly washed, teeth should be brushed
and flossed, and genitals should be clean. The hands and genitals
are especially important—the hands because they fondle the
genital openings, which are a clean part of the body that become
infected when exposed to germs, and the genitals because they
can easily become contaminated by feces from the rectum. When
freshly washed and free of infection, the genitals are clean.

How does a woman stimulate a man so he is prepared for entry by her invitation?

The woman's invitation for entry should not be a demand
that the man must be ready at that moment. It just means
that whenever he is ready, she is. Often, if the woman is
ready, her arousal will have gotten the man eager too. The
woman participates in preparing the man for entry, not only
by her own involvement and responsiveness, but also by
enjoying her husband's genitals. Stroking the shaft of the
penis, in addition to enjoying his entire body, will usually get
a man ready for entry.

Do most women experience bleeding and pain when the hymen breaks during the first entry?

The response can range from absolutely no pain and no bleeding to such severe pain that entry is impossible and there is noticeable bleeding. The last two possibilities are rare. When the vaginal opening has been stretched and a lubricant is used, and when the women guides the penis in at her own pace, there is often no bleeding and only a momentary "Ouch!"

What can I do to reduce my fear of the pain of intercourse? I am a virgin and I am dreading the wedding night.

Unfortunately, your *fear* is likely to cause pain unless you work past it. The fear will not go away by ignoring it. Talk about it, and prepare, prepare, prepare! Stretch your vaginal opening at least twenty minutes daily. Get a gynecological examination, and ask your physician for dilators. Learn to control your PC muscle so you can voluntarily relax it. Learn visualization and relaxation techniques. Every day when you stretch your vagina, picture your first sexual intercourse. Note when your fear sets in. Replace the fear with positive thoughts and feelings. Imagine the penis in your vagina feeling like a warm, soft, moist, loving sensation. Take charge of when and how entry happens. Use lots of lubricant. Let your husband know as soon as you feel afraid. Stop pursuing entry at that point and just hold and affirm one another, then try again. Often anticipation is the biggest hurdle. Once you actually pursue entry, the fears may dissipate. If you cannot get beyond your fear, get help from a sexual therapist.

What if my wife is initially aroused and then loses lubrication before entry?

This is very common. That is why we recommend using a lubricant every time until you notice you have forgotten to use it. Lubrication occurs within ten to twenty seconds of any genital stimulation. During prolonged love play, lubrication is likely to dry.

Must a woman have an orgasm every time?

Some women feel a need for an orgasm every time; others do not. There is no right or wrong. The woman's enjoyment of the sexual experience may have nothing to do with having an orgasm. For her it may be the closeness and connection that is most satisfying. This varies greatly from woman to woman. A successful sexual experience is not dependent upon arousal, orgasm, ejaculation, or intercourse.

Isn't it uncomfortable for the woman to lead?

It depends on how she leads. If she is controlling, demeaning, or demanding, it is very uncomfortable. If she sets the pace by being open about what she is feeling and desiring and her husband sensitively responds to her, it can be wonderful for both. The woman is more variable and complex in her need for emotional readiness, her physical responsiveness, and her sexual desires than the man is. Because of this, it usually works best if the man delights in the woman but lets her set the pace.

If a woman is experienced and her husband is not, it will be very important for her to lead until they are equally comfortable with the sexual activity.

It seems like after waiting so long for sex, we're going to want to go right to sexual intercourse on our wedding night. Is it detrimental to go right from foreplay to intercourse without getting acquainted with each other's genitals?

Getting acquainted with each other's genitals, even though it seems like that would be beneficial to do before pursuing sexual intercourse, is likely to feel rather clinical and exposing for a newly married couple. Even couples who have been married for years sometimes have difficulty being that vulnerable with each other. We don't think that would be a necessary step to consummating your marriage. It is natural on the wedding night to just let down all restrictions and go for it. Do be sure to include the conditions described previously for a "successful" wedding-night experience so you don't move too quickly from foreplay to intercourse and feel let down.

8 KEEP THE SPARK ALIVE

Shifting from your premarital romantic or passion-driven sexual energy to a deeper, more intimate, and long-lasting sexual relationship will keep your sexual spark alive throughout your marriage. To do that, you will need to counteract the myth that satisfying sex will just happen naturally. The quality of your sexual relationship is not dependent upon fate; it is dependent upon *you*.

DEVELOP A POSITIVE SEXUAL CONFIDENCE

Sexual self-confidence has to be learned. The general self-confidence you gained or lacked during your childhood years will either help or hinder your sexual self-confidence. If you lack general self-confidence, you will need to develop good feelings about yourself as a person before you will be able to enjoy sex with confidence.

Knowledge, practice, and positive sexual experiences will lead you to a positive sexual confidence that will allow you to know your sexual needs and desires without being demanding or insecure in pursuing those needs with your spouse. Sexual self-confidence is a quiet, inner sexual awareness that can let you enjoy the giving and receiving of sexual pleasure, without insisting on sex for satisfaction. If you are secure in your sexuality, you will accept each other's sexual differences and not take them as a personal assault of your sexual attractiveness. Thus, your sexual self-confidence will enable you to keep sex for mutual pleasure in your marriage.

NURTURE INDIVIDUAL AND RELATIONSHIP GROWTH

A relationship is only as strong as the individuals who join together to form it. A sexual relationship is only as dynamic as the general relationship of the two who are sharing their bodies with each other. The two of you will need to allow separateness, as well as plan for quality togetherness. Attend to personal and relationship needs as they arise. If you don't, those issues will eventually spill over into the bedroom. As the two of you learn to bring out the best in each other, you will each become better individuals, and your relationship will grow deeper in love and in sexual enjoyment.

LEARN TO PLEASURE EACH OTHER FOR THE SAKE OF PLEASURE

To focus on pleasure in your sexual relationship, you will need to bring to your marriage or develop the attitude that you have the *right* to pleasure, and so does your spouse. Both of you are worthy of sexual pleasure, but you will only be able to give and receive pleasure freely if each of you feels free from sexual demands. Anxiety due to demands you give yourselves or each other will interfere with every phase of the sexual experience.

To keep your sexual experiences focused on pleasure and free of demands, begin each sexual time with the reminder that you are there to enjoy yourselves and each other without any demand to have to get aroused, to have to perform for each other in any certain way, to have to be orgasmic, or to have to have intercourse. Lovemaking is the time for the two of you to pull away from all the demands and responsibilities of life and just delight in each other without any expectations—never by violating the other person. The only expectation is that you give your bodies to each other for mutual pleasure. Pleasure cannot be demanded, but rather, is freely pursued.

The involuntary responses of sexual arousal and release may occur when you are relaxed and soaking in sexual pleasure, but they cannot be the goal. When you *try* to get aroused or *try* to have an orgasm, your trying will interfere with those natural bodily responses. If you find yourself trying, distract yourself by telling your spouse that you are demanding a response of yourself. Verbalizing your mental demands and anxieties will distract you from them and help you refocus on the good sensations of touching and being touched.

Focusing on pleasure enhances your bodily awareness by letting you soak in the sensuous touch and skin-to-skin contact of each other's body. This works best when each of you is able to give your body to each other to enjoy and able to enjoy each other's body.

KEEP KISSING

Kissing is the most intimate form of pleasuring; make sure it is a positive part of lovemaking for both of you. That may be difficult to talk about, especially if one of you is not pleased with how the other kisses. To express corrections can be very hurtful, yet it is vital that the two of you learn to mutually enjoy passionate kissing. To do that, we recommend that you first talk about any past negative experiences either of you have had with kissing. If kissing was ever forced on you abusively, it will be important that you lead in all kissing until you are able to invite kisses from your spouse. Then take turns leading and teaching each other how you like to kiss. Experiment with new ways. Kissing is an indicator of a sexual relationship. It is rare for a couple with sexual difficulties to say they enjoy their kissing. If you keep kissing alive, your sexual relationship is likely to also do well. Kissing keeps the pilot light on so that it won't be difficult to turn up the flame!

PURSUE SEXUAL PLEASURE RESPONSIBLY

Not only do each of you have equal rights to sexual pleasure in marriage, you also have equal responsibility. Enjoying each other's body and letting each event take on its own character is easiest when each of you feels comfortable pursuing your own desire for touch. As both pleasurer and receiver, you must take responsibility for discovering, communicating, and going after your sexual feelings and needs, but never at the other's expense.

Your sex life will continue to sizzle when you are both fully enjoying yourselves sexually, and able to freely give and receive pleasure. As the receiver of touch, your only task is to soak in the pleasure and to redirect your spouse when the touch is not pleasing. You can check with your spouse if at any time you think your pleasure may be interfering with his or her pleasure. As the pleasurer, your only responsibility is to lovingly touch your spouse in a way that feels good to you, enjoying his or her body for your pleasure. Caress slowly. Take time to radiate warmth through your fingertips and to take in the sensation and pulsation of your spouse's body. You cannot expect your spouse to know when, how, and where you want to be pleasured; you are responsible to let each other know your needs and desires. This only works if that is a mutual commitment.

ANTICIPATE YOUR SEXUAL TIMES

As with anything else in life, *timing* and *anticipation* are important ingredients to keeping the spark alive. If you have set aside blocks of time to be available to each other physically, you will be able to mentally picture and prepare yourselves for your times together. If quality time has not been predetermined, you can anticipate and find time for your sexual relationship by constantly picturing the two of you together and enjoying bodily pleasure. Your ongoing positive expectation of having time together will work well.

CULTIVATE ROMANCE

Pay attention to those little details of your sexual relationship that will add romance. Romance will help you shift from initial passion to an ongoing life of sexual fulfillment. Continue to woo, court, and seduce each other. Pay attention to your spouse. Touch each other when you pass by. Take a moment to give your spouse a positive message of regard and care. Write notes of affection and appreciation to each other, and withhold unkind thoughts and feelings.

Create a romantic atmosphere that appeals to all the senses: sight, smell, touch, sound, and even taste. If your living situation will allow for it, design your bedroom or your most common lovemaking location to have a sense of separateness to which you can escape. Enhance your lovemaking atmosphere by keeping it free of clutter and add touches that each of you enjoy. Music is often a great addition. You may enjoy moving your bodies together to the rhythm of the music. Dancing in the nude in the privacy of your bedroom can be a romantic beginning to sharing your bodies with each other. A dimmer switch on the light, a colored light bulb, or candlelight are all possible visual variations. Privacy is a necessity. The first item of repair when you move into a new home should be a lock on the bedroom door!

Romance does not have to be fervent or serious; it can also be fun. Lighten up in the ways you express romance. Be adventurous and childlike. A little tease can add spark to your romantic life. You both need to have a sense of humor for teasing to work effectively, and the teasing must not be hurtful or degrading in any way. It has to be fun and uplifting for both of you. Romance will slip away if you do not consciously decide to keep it alive.

KEEP THE LINES OF COMMUNICATION OPEN

Bernie Zilbergeld, in *The New Male Sexuality*, gives a delightful description of how couples can establish openness about their sexual relationship:

> This is what I think of as oral sex: opening one's mouth and saying something. Every survey I'm aware of has found a strong positive correlation between this and sexual satisfaction. It's not that people who have good sex over time always talk about it or even that they talk about it a lot. It's simply that they have the option of talking about sex when there's something to be said.[1]

Your ability and willingness to talk about sex will depend upon the naturalness and ease with which you are able to share your thoughts, desires, feelings, and fantasies about your sexual relationship as they arise. Some couples need to schedule times to talk, sort of like you schedule a six-month checkup for your car.

ELIMINATE HINDRANCES TO SUCCESS

Throughout this book, we've referred directly or indirectly to the hindrances to a positive, fulfilling sexual relationship in marriage. As a review, we'll provide a summary here. We believe the items on this list are self-explanatory. Getting your sex life off to a great start means you are aware of these possible problems and you know how to avoid them.

Sex is too quick.

Sex is functional and for physical release only.

Sex is a substitute for intimacy rather than an expression of intimacy.

Either or both of the spouses are trying to please each other rather than delight in each other.

Either or both have come to the marriage with unresolved sexual issues from the past.

Either or both come with unrealistic sexual expectations.

Relationship conflicts need to be resolved.

Sex becomes mechanical and a matter of routine.

Sex only happens when both or one is fatigued; quality time is not allowed for sex.

Sex means simply arousal, release, and/or intercourse.

Sex is one-sided rather than a mutual expression designed for mutual fulfillment.

When Pain Interrupts Pleasure

Sex is meant to feel good. When sex hurts, its purpose is interrupted. Thus, pain during intercourse must be taken very seriously and relief sought with diligence.

Vaginismus. The involuntary, spastic contracting of the muscles surrounding the entrance to the vagina can make penetration extremely painful or impossible. This problem results from negative feelings such as fear, pain, and violation that have been connected with vaginal penetration or the anticipation of it.

You can learn to relax the tightened vaginal muscle by working through one or more of the following four tracks: (1) Through reading, writing, and talking, you can free yourself of the emotional conflict and tension associated with entry into the vagina. (2) Through a sexual-retraining process, you can learn to trust the giving and receiving of sexual pleasure. (3) You can engage in an active process to help you gain acceptance of and voluntary control over your genitals. (4) You can achieve entry into the vagina through a gradual process of reducing fear and relaxing the vaginal opening. The last step is the most unique to this particular problem; vaginal dilation exercises are the key to successful treatment of vaginismus.

Entry into the vagina without pain can be achieved without surgery or other intrusive procedures. You *can* learn to control that muscle so that entry does not cause pain.

Physically Based Pain. An increasing number of women, particularly young women, are reporting pain during intercourse. Pain does not have to be tolerated. In fact, pain cannot be allowed to continue if you are going to enjoy sexual pleasure. Several physical problems can cause pain during intercourse: Infections, irritations, tears or fissures, childbirth trauma, or a tipped uterus are some of the most common. To reduce physically based pain, follow these guidelines:

1. Talk with your husband about the pain. Develop a signal

to let him know when you are feeling pain so you can change your activity to relieve it. Any sexual activity associated with pain should never be continued.

2. Identify exactly *when* in your sexual experience the pain is triggered and *how long* it lasts. Note specifically *where* the pain is located. It is helpful if you can describe *what type of pain* you experience: stinging, burning, stabbing, dull, rubbing, or sharp.

3. Take charge of getting relief from your pain. Seek medical help and describe in detail what you have already discovered about your pain. Boldly inform your physician that the pain is interrupting your sexual pleasure, and you want treatment to relieve that pain. If the physician minimizes your pain or tells you to just keep trying, change physicians!

4. Enjoy and focus on the sexual activities that do not elicit pain.

NURTURE THE EMOTIONAL-RELATIONSHIP DIMENSION OF SEX

The key ingredients of your sexual relationship must be attended to if you are going to keep your sexual spark alive. These ingredients that we discussed in chapter 2 are sexual desire, initiation, pleasuring, letting go, and affirming.

Sexual Desire

Sexual desire is the urge to be touched, to be close, or it is the urge for sexual arousal, orgasm, or intercourse. Sexual desire is God-given and innate in every one, even though that desire is experienced differently by different people.

For some, sexual interest has a very natural ebb and flow throughout life that may occur spontaneously and automatically. If that is true for you, your desire may surface somewhat regularly according to the buildup of sexual energy, or it may occur as you exercise or pamper your body. It may be set off by a certain expression, look, activity, or talent, or by seeing or touching each other. Sexual desire may get started by something sensuous, like music, the sound of ocean waves, a romantic setting, a scent, a story, or a picture.

Others do not seem to have that automatic awareness of sexual desire. You may need certain conditions to make you aware of those needs. You may become aware of sexual urges when you are away from the pressures of life—your work, your children, or social obligations.

Having a special time for each other may trigger your sexual desire: a private time at home in your bedroom, a special meal together, a time of talking together, or a time of physical, emotional, or spiritual connection.

There may be very specific behaviors that ignite your sexual urges, actions you do yourself or behaviors you need from your spouse. You may need a hug, a kiss, help with the chores, or an action that says, "I care about you." It may be that you need to take time to prepare yourself mentally by thinking about being together sexually (that positive mental anticipation we talked about earlier in this chapter) or by reading something romantic.

When you need a specific behavior from your spouse to spark your sexual interest, getting what you need becomes more complicated. Sex works best in all dimensions when each of you takes responsibility for your own needs. Therefore, when your need requires action by your spouse, you must communicate that need. Avoid the game of thinking, *If he loves me, he'll know what I need. I've told him before, so he should remember. If I have to tell him, it won't work.* If you convince yourself it won't work, it surely won't. So take responsibility to know and communicate clearly, openly, and consistently what you need to activate your sexual urges.

Initiation

Acting on your sexual desire with one another is initiation. You may initiate sexual contact before any arousal or as the result of being turned on or sexually excited. Initiation may be the expression of your desire to just be close and warm, or for intense sexual play that will lead to intercourse and release. It may grow mutually between the two of you, or it may come from one of you to the other. Mutual initiation often grows out of physical contact like a hug, a kiss, or crawling into bed together. Spending time working, playing, talking, or just being together may also spark desire that triggers mutual pursuit of sexual behavior.

More often initiation occurs when one sexually desirous spouse expresses desire for the other. This interest may be communicated in words, by reaching out physically, or in more subtle ways. The message may be a direct, verbal invitation or a more symbolic message. You will likely develop your own love language to express desire to be with one another sexually. Many women need their husbands to express their desire as positive messages about them or as messages of their value to the husbands. Women respond much more favorably to "You are gorgeous. I'd love to spend some time with you" than to "I need sex" or "You haven't met my sexual needs in a long time." The last two requests make the woman feel like she could be anyone, as long as she gives him an ejaculation. She feels as if she is servicing him. A physical approach works great if it is positive for both, but if one of you feels that hugs or kisses are given only to "get sex," that can cause you to avoid those wonderful expressions of affection. Physical initiation must be an expression of care and connection with each other without a demand from one spouse to the other. Subtle initiation is fun if the other one catches the subtleties. Preparing your body, the setting, or a special treat are all possible subtle ways to initiate sex.

Initiation flows best and causes the least amount of tension when both of you are free to express your desires without putting pressure on the other to feel the same as you do or to respond with enthusiasm. If the other does not feel open to a sexual encounter, an option other than "no" should be offered. You make yourselves vulnerable when you express your desire for each other. Getting a "no" as a response can hurt. A more positive response might be, "Boy, you caught me off guard. Give me a little time to see if I can get with that possibility." You could also offer other options: "I'm exhausted, but what if I get to bed early and we set the alarm to have some time tomorrow morning?" or "I don't have the energy to get aroused, but I would love some pleasuring, and I wouldn't mind bringing you as far as you'd like." The possibilities are endless. They could include a later time, a different physical activity, or a different focus. Almost anything is better than "no."

Pleasuring

Becoming one—totally—takes time. It takes time to mesh your worlds, communicate with one another, and delight in the stimulation of each other's body. Pleasuring begins with the process of getting into each other's world and bringing together your emotions, spirits, sensations, and bodies. It includes a focus on all of the senses. You must both appeal to each other's needs for sight, smell, touch, sound, and taste. Meshing will occur more naturally when you have spent time together; it will take more effort if your worlds have been separate and consuming.

Two types of communication are necessary to enjoy pleasuring: verbal and nonverbal. Talking about what you like, don't like, or would like should be done apart from the sexual experience. Verbal messages during sex should indicate your enjoyment and express positive invitations for the touch you would enjoy. Nonverbal communication lets you signal each other during sex without interrupting the flow of the pleasure. These nonverbal signals can be taught apart from the sexual experience.

Delighting in the erotic touching of each other's body is vital to the giving and receiving of pleasure and will likely trigger some arousal and possibly release. To maximize the pleasure each of you receives, acknowledge your body's hunger for touch and go after that, enjoy touching each other in ways that are pleasurable to you, and agree to let each other know if any activity is negative by inviting some other touch that would feel better. Since women are more complex and sensitive, it usually works best if the woman sets the pace for sexual stimulation. As one woman explained to her husband, "It's like when we ride bikes together. Since you can go faster than I can, it works best if you always keep your front tire right behind mine." Sex often works best if the husband thinks of keeping his activity and intensity just a little behind her. A sexually satisfied woman is usually one who has taught her husband how and when she wants to be stimulated sexually. That requires a husband who is willing to learn from his wife and allow her to be the expert on her body.

Being able to love each other and enjoy erotic touching without feeling the need to please, without demanding performance, and without feeling failure is vital to a delightful, lifelong sexual relationship.

Entry

Total sexual union is not necessary to have total sexual fulfillment or the intimacy of bodily pleasure. As we have said repeatedly, when entry of the penis into the vagina is desired, it is best if it is initiated by the woman since it is her body that is being entered. We all feel threatened or violated when someone enters our "territory" without being invited. Thus, it will relax you, the woman, to know that your husband will wait for you to signal him when you are ready for entry. It will also take the pressure off him to magically know when you want entry.

Enjoying the Process

Entry of the penis into the vagina does not have to be the beginning of the end. When the focus is on pleasuring rather than orgasm, there can be a time of resting together and enjoying the penetration of the penis into the vagina without thrusting. There can be freedom to withdraw, reenter, and "play around," allowing the turned-on feelings to ebb and flow in intensity. This is the time in the sexual experience to abandon all fears and inhibitions so you are free to intensify the heavy breathing, rhythmic movement, noises, and grimaces that are a natural part of the body's sexual response to pleasure.

When you are both able to enjoy the process and let sex flow freely, the moods of your sexual experiences will tend to vary from tenderness to passion to fun and games. Sometimes the mood may be intensely erotic and at other times functional. Either can be a pleasurable way to meet your sexual needs.

Letting Go

When you are not controlled or inhibited and you are receiving adequate stimulation, letting go will occur somewhere in the process of lovemaking. Letting go is obvious in men but may be a struggle or a source of confusion for many women.

To help women understand the sensation of letting go, we compare it to a sneeze. The buildup of tension in the pelvis is due to vasocongestion—blood and fluid filling the genitals—just like the nasal passages get congested before a sneeze. There is that tingling sensation both in the nose before a sneeze and in the pelvis before an orgasm. You can stop an orgasm just like you can stop a sneeze, but you cannot "will" either to happen. If those pelvic, tingling sensations are pursued with stimulation and activity, the contractions in the passageways will release the tension and fullness—that is an orgasm, a pelvic sneeze!

Affirmation

When you allow yourselves to be vulnerable and let go sexually—to be out of control and release all of your sexual intensity with one another—a closeness and a deep sense of warmth follow. This is an important time of sharing. When you have not been able to let go of all the intensity that built up during sexual arousal, you may feel tense or frustrated or disappointed. We encourage you to continue your closeness during the crying, if that happens. Hold each other rather than pulling away. Affirm your love, care, and commitment to each other.

Learning to keep sex for pleasure is vital to making the transition from a passion-driven sexual relationship to an ongoing sexual relationship. Once two people can have each other every day and there are no restrictions on their being together sexually, sex changes. There is something that happens when two individuals become one and commit themselves to each other for a lifetime. Turn that change into incredible freedom!

As you establish positive sexual patterns, eliminate hindrances to success, and attend to the emotional-relationship dimensions of sex early in your married sex life, you will set a positive tone for years of sexual enjoyment with each other. You can enjoy sex with increasing vigor for the rest of your married life—and that would be our hope for you. May your affection, love, and enjoyment of each other's body continue to soar year after year.

NOTES

Chapter 2: Clarify Expectations

1. Nowval Geldenhuys, B.A., B.D., Th.M., *The Intimate Life* (Grand Rapids: Eerdmans, 1957), 36.
2. James Dobson, *Love for a Lifetime: Building a Marriage That Will Go the Distance* (Portland: Multnomah, 1987), 44.
3. John Gray, *Men Are from Mars, Women Are from Venus* (New York: HarperCollins, 1993).

Chapter 3: Know Your Body

1. Adapted from Masters and Johnson, *Human Sexual Response* (Boston: Little, Brown & Co., 1966).
2. Alan P. Brauer and Donna J. Brauer, *ESO* (New York: Warner, 2001), chapter 6.
3. Julia R. Heiman and Joseph LoPiccolo, *Becoming Orgasmic* (New York: Prentice Hall, 1992).
4. Clifford Penner and Joyce Penner, *Restoring the Pleasure* (Dallas: Word, 1993).

Chapter 5: Prepare for Your First Time

1. Paul Popenoe, Sc.D., *Preparing for Marriage* (Los Angeles: American Institute of Family Relations, 1938; reprint 1961).
2. Ibid., 5.
3. Helen Singer Kaplan, *PE: How to Overcome Premature Ejaculation* (New York: Brunner/Mazel, 1979).

4. Michael E. Metz, Ph.D. and Barry McCarthy, *Coping with Premature Ejaculation: How to Overcome PE, Please Your Partner, & Have Great Sex* (Oakland: New Harbinger, 2004).

Chapter 6: Family-Planning Options

1. Birth Control Guide: http://www.fda.gov.
2. Birth Control Guide: http://www.fda.gov.
3. Birth Control Guide: http://www.fda.gov.
4. *Contraceptive Technology,* 17th ed. (New York: Irvington Publishers, 1994), 113, 154.
5. Birth Control Guide: http://www.fda.gov.
6. Fact Sheets: Intrauterine Devices: http://www.cdc.gov, October 24, 2003.
7. *Contraceptive Technology,* 113.
8. Ibid., 348.
9. Ibid., 113.
10. Richard P. Dickey, M.D., Ph.D., *Managing Contraceptive Pill Patients,* 11th ed. (Durant, Okla.: Essential Medical Systems, 2002).
11. Ibid., 82–83.
12. *Contraceptive Technology,* 272–75.
13. Ibid., 274.
14. Ibid., 288.
15. Birth Control Guide: http://www.fda.gov.
16. John J. Billings, *The Ovulation Method: Natural Family Planning* (Collegeville, MN: Liturgical Press, 1992).

Chapter 8: Keep the Spark Alive

1. Bernie Zilbergeld, *The New Male Sexuality* (New York: Bantam, 1999), 353.

ADDITIONAL REFERENCES

Berman, Jennifer, Laura Berman, and Elisabeth Bumiller. *For Women Only: A Revolutionary Guide to Overcoming Sexual Dysfunction and Reclaiming Your Sex Life*. New York: Henry Holt and Company, 2001.

Chapman, Gary. *The Five Love Languages*. Chicago: Northfield Publishing, 1992.

Cobb, Nancy, and Connie Grigsby. *The Best Thing I Ever Did for My Marriage: 50 Real-Life Stories*. Sisters, OR: Multnomah, 2003.

Dillow, Linda, and Lorraine Pintus. *Intimate Issues: 21 Questions Christian Women Ask About Sex*. Colorado Springs, CO: Waterbrook Press, 1999.

Dobson, James C. *Love for a Lifetime: Building a Marriage That Will Go the Distance*. Portland: Multnomah, 1987.

Foley, Sallie, Sally A. Kope, and Dennis P. Sugrue. *Sex Matters for Women: A Complete Guide to Taking Care of Your Sexual Self*. New York: Guilford Press, 2002.

Godek, Gregory J. P. *1001 Ways to Be Romantic*. Naperville, IL: Casablanca Press, 1999.

Laaser, Mark. *Faithful and True*. Grand Rapids: Zondervan, 1996.

———. *L.I.F.E. Guide for Men*. Longwood, FL: Xulon Press, 2002.

McCarthy, Barry. *Male Sexual Awareness*. New York: Carroll and Graf, 1988.

McCarthy, Barry, and Emily McCarthy. *Couple Sexual Awareness*. New York: Carroll and Graf, 1998.

————. *Female Sexual Awareness.* New York: Carroll and Graf, 1989.

McIlhaney, Joe S., Jr., M.D. *1250 Health-Care Questions Women Ask.* Grand Rapids: Baker, 1992.

Parrott, Les, and Leslie Parrott. *Becoming Soul Mates.* Grand Rapids: Zondervan, 1997.

————. *Pillow Talk for Couples: Drawing Closer Before the Lights Go Out.* Nashville: J. Countryman, 2003.

————. *Saving Your Marriage Before It Starts: Seven Questions to Ask Before (and After) You Marry.* Grand Rapids: Zondervan, 1995.

Penner, Clifford, and Joyce Penner. *The Gift of Sex.* Nashville: W Publishing Group, 2003.

————. *The Married Guy's Guide to Great Sex.* Carol Stream, IL: Tyndale, 2004.

————. *Sex Facts for the Family.* Dallas: Word, 1992.

Schnarch, David M., Ph.D. *Constructing the Sexual Crucible: An Integration of Sexual and Marital Therapy.* New York: Norton, 1991.

Smalley, Gary, and John Trent, Ph.D. *The Language of Love.* Colorado Springs, CO: Focus on the Family, 1991.

Smedes, Lewis B. *Forgive and Forget: Healing the Hurts We Don't Deserve.* San Francisco: Harper & Row, 1984.

————. *Sex for Christians.* Grand Rapids: Eerdmans, 1994.

Warren, Neil Clark. *Finding the Love of Your Life.* Colorado Springs, CO: Focus on the Family, 1992.

Wright, Norman H. *So You're Getting Married.* Ventura, CA: Regal Books, 1985.

ABOUT THE AUTHORS

DR. CLIFFORD AND JOYCE PENNER are internationally recognized sexual therapists, educators, and authors. Joyce, a registered nurse and clinical nurse specialist, holds a B.S. in nursing from the University of Washington and a master's degree in psychosomatic nursing and nursing education from UCLA. Clifford, a clinical psychologist, earned an M.A. in theology from Fuller Theological Seminary and holds a Ph.D. from Fuller's Graduate School of Psychology. The Penners have authored nine books, including *The Gift of Sex, Restoring the Pleasure, Getting Your Sex Life Off to a Great Start,* and *The Married Guy's Guide to Great Sex.* In addition to conducting sex education and sexual enhancement seminars, they maintain a full-time practice in sexual therapy in Pasadena, California.